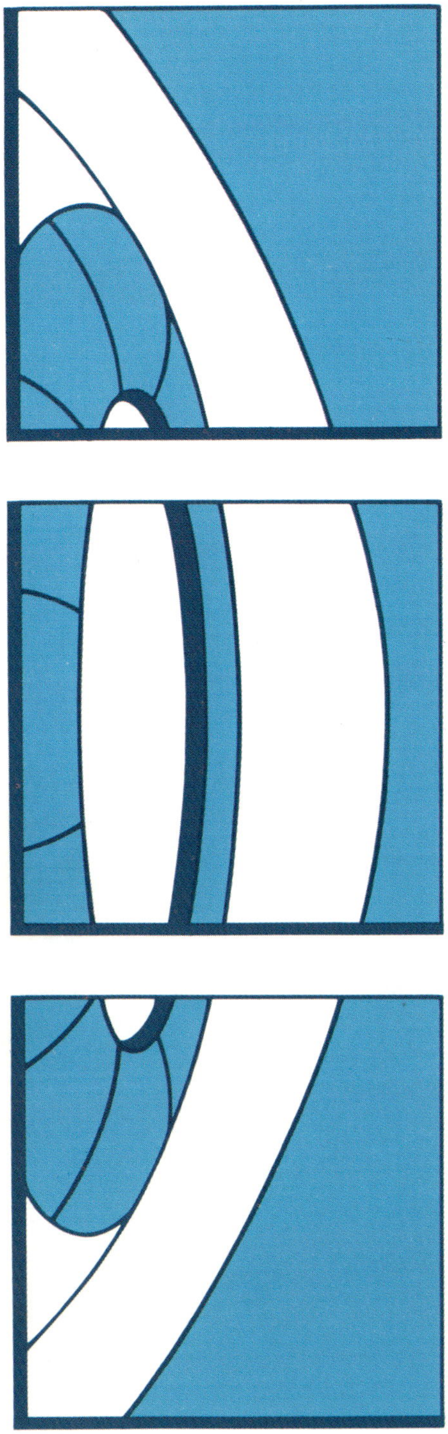

Eric R. Mandel, M.D.
Lenox Hill Hospital,
Cornea and External Disease,
New York, New York

Clinical Fellow in Ophthalmology,
Cornea and External Disease Service,
Massachusetts Eye and Ear Infirmary,
Boston, Massachusetts

Michael D. Wagoner, M.D.
Assistant Professor of Ophthalmology,
Harvard Medical School
Cornea and External Disease Service,
Massachusetts Eye and Ear Infirmary
Boston, Massachusetts

Atlas of Corneal Disease

1989
W. B. SAUNDERS COMPANY
Harcourt Brace Jovanovich, Inc.

Philadelphia □ London □ Toronto
Montreal □ Sydney □ Tokyo

W. B. SAUNDERS COMPANY
Harcourt Brace Jovanovich, Inc.

The Curtis Center
Independence Square West
Philadelphia, PA 19106

Library of Cc ress Cataloging-in-Publication Data
Mandel, Eric K
Atlas of corneal disease.
1. Cornea—Diseases—Atlases. I. Wagoner, Michael D. II. Title.
[DNLM: 1. Corneal Diseases—atlases. WW 17 M271a]
RE336.M35 1989 617.7′19 88–15817
ISBN 0-7216-2160-0

Editor: Lisa McAllister
Designer: W. B. Saunders Staff
Production Manager: Carolyn Naylor
Manuscript Editor: RoseMarie Klimowicz
Cover Designer: Arlette Ramphal
Illustration Coordinator: Lisa Lambert
Indexer: Kathleen Garcia

Atlas of Corneal Disease ISBN 0–7216–2160–0

Last digit is the print number: 9 8 7 6 5 4 3 2 1

This book is dedicated to our families.

Contributors

Mark B. Abelson, MD Assistant Clinical Professor, Department of Ophthalmology, Harvard Medical School, Cornea Service, Massachusetts Eye and Ear Infirmary, Boston, Massachusetts

S. Arthur Boruchoff, MD Associate Clinical Professor, Department of Ophthalmology, Harvard Medical School, Cornea Service, Massachusetts Eye and Ear Infirmary, Boston, Massachusetts

Claes H. Dohlman, MD Professor and Chairman, Department of Ophthalmology, Harvard Medical School, Cornea Service, Massachusetts Eye and Ear Infirmary, Boston, Massachusetts

C. Stephen Foster, MD Associate Professor, Department of Ophthalmology, Harvard Medical School; Director, Uveitis Service and Hilles Laboratory of Immunology, Cornea Service, Massachusetts Eye and Ear Infirmary, Boston, Massachusetts

Jeffrey P. Gilbard, MD Assistant Professor, Department of Ophthalmology, Harvard Medical School; Cornea Service, Massachusetts Eye and Ear Infirmary, Boston, Massachusetts

Kenneth R. Kenyon, MD Associate Professor, Department of Ophthalmology, Harvard Medical School; Director, Cornea Service, Massachusetts Eye and Ear Infirmary, Boston, Massachusetts

Deborah Pavan-Langston, MD Associate Professor, Department of Ophthalmology, Harvard Medical School, Cornea Service, Massachusetts Eye and Ear Infirmary, Boston, Massachusetts

Roger F. Steinert, MD Assistant Clinical Professor, Department of Ophthalmology, Harvard Medical School, Cornea Service, Massachusetts Eye and Ear Infirmary, Boston, Massachusetts

Richard A. Thoft, MD Chairman, Department of Ophthalmology, The Eye and Ear Institute, University of Pittsburgh, Pittsburgh, Pennsylvania

Michael D. Wagoner, MD Assistant Professor, Department of Ophthalmology, Harvard Medical School, Cornea Service, Massachusetts Eye and Ear Infirmary, Boston, Massachusetts

Preface

The purpose of this book is to provide a detailed, photographic supplement to the excellent, comprehensive textbooks of corneal disease that are already available. The legends are purely descriptive and do not attempt to duplicate or substitute for detailed discussions, which can be found in other authoritative volumes. It is hoped that this format will be useful both to introduce the medical student and nonophthalmic practitioner to the field of corneal disease, and at the same time to provide a source of review and reference for the ophthalmic resident and practitioner.

We have endeavored to cover comprehensively the entire spectrum of corneal disease as well as other ophthalmic or systemic disorders with associated corneal findings. Of necessity, many lid and conjunctival diseases with limited significance for the cornea have been excluded. Some topics that are not part of our collective experience have not been included. While an effort has been made to balance the presentation of classic and nonclassic appearances, the spectrum of severity, and the natural history of the selected topics, it is clear that the subspecialty interests of the contributing authors have often resulted in detailed attention to "esoteric" conditions. Rather than regard this as a weakness or flaw, we feel that this permits us to include more detail on selected subjects (e.g., ocular cicatricial pemphigoid, alkali injuries) than is present in any single previously published work. These disproportionate exhibitions are not done at the expense of inclusion of the more commonly encountered corneal diseases, and the space devoted to each topic is not meant to reflect our bias regarding relative importance.

For the purpose of convenience the book has been divided into nine chapters, each covering a broad general category. Clearly, no single classification system can ever be completely satisfactory, since many diseases (e.g., Mooren's ulceration) do not readily lend themselves to our classification system. Certain topics have been represented in multiple sections. For example, infectious diseases are covered both in the chapter devoted to this topic and among the complications of corneal surgery. Similarly, while no sections are devoted to the descriptive diagnosis "sterile corneal ulceration" or "peripheral ulcerative keratititis," examples of these can be found under the specific etiologic disorder that has produced this appearance. Finally, morphologic changes common to many corneal diseases (e.g., corneal vascularization, corneal wound healing) are not covered separately but are extensively represented throughout the book wherever they occur in association with a specific condition.

We apologize for any inaccuracies, omissions, or inconsistencies and welcome helpful criticisms and suggestions. We hope you will find the photographs useful and enjoy them as much as we enjoyed selecting and putting them together.

Eric Mandel, MD
Michael D. Wagoner, MD

Acknowledgments

This book could not have been possible without the collective effort of many individuals. First, and foremost, we must recognize the collective effort of all the members of the Cornea Service of the Massachusetts Eye and Ear Infirmary of this decade who unselfishly made their entire slide collections and patient records available for consideration for inclusion in this volume. For their efforts they are each recognized equally as contributing authors to this volume. We would also like to thank our outstanding ophthalmic photographer, Philip H. Ruderman, who performed most of the photographic work in this volume and therefore had a direct impact on the quality of the book. Finally, a special word of thanks should be extended to Dr. Claes Dohlman, founder of the Cornea Service, for his unsurpassed teaching ability and encouragement to initiate and complete this book.

Eric Mandel, MD
Michael Wagoner, MD

Contents

1

Corneal Dystrophies

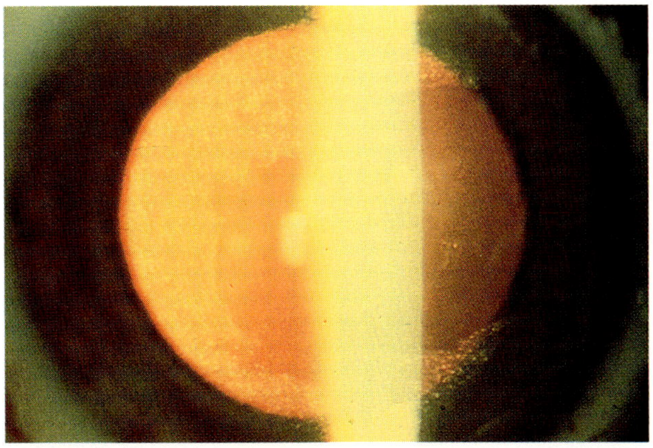

Juvenile hereditary epithelial dystrophy (Meesman's dystrophy).

Figure 1–1. Multiple tiny, round, clear vesicles in a crescentic limbal pattern are seen in the corneal epithelium with retroillumination.

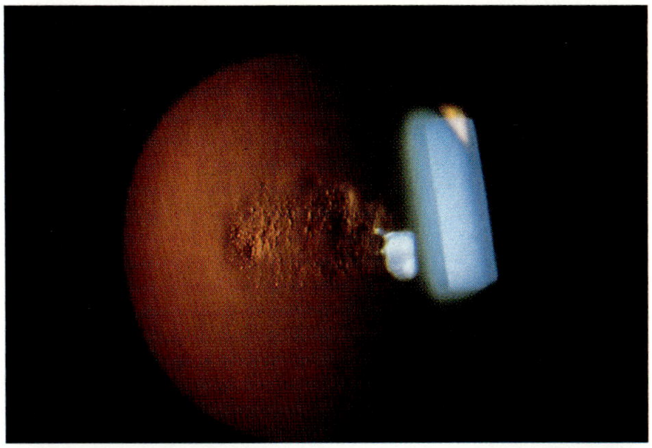

Juvenile hereditary epithelial dystrophy (Meesman's dystrophy).

Figure 1–2. Multiple intraepithelial vesicles are present in the typical interpalpebral distribution.

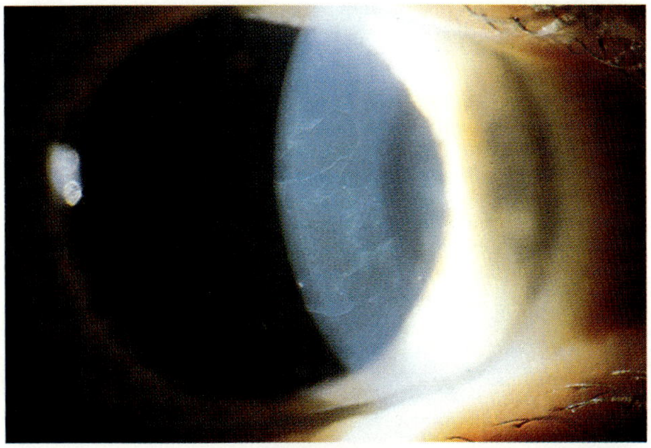

Epithelial basement membrane dystrophy (map-dot-fingerprint dystrophy, Cogan's dystrophy).

Figure 1–3. A diffuse gray lesion with a clear, oval center resembling a map is seen temporal to the visual axis. No other areas are involved.

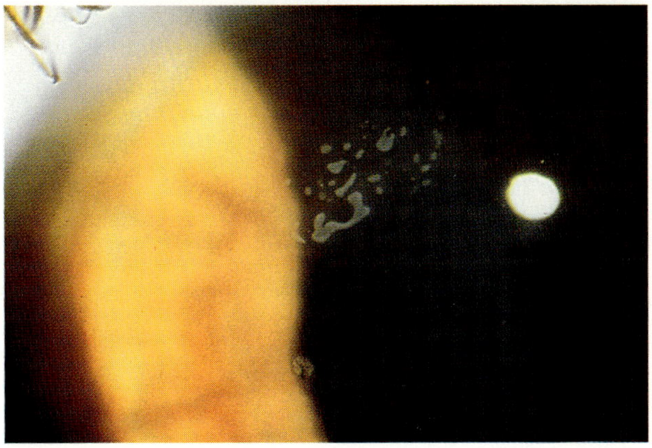

Epithelial basement membrane dystrophy.

Figure 1–4. Multiple gray, well-circumscribed lesions resembling dots of varying size are clustered in one region of the cornea.

Epithelial basement membrane dystrophy.

Figure 1–5. Multiple refractile, "fingerprint" lines are seen with retroillumination. (Courtesy of Dr. Lawrence Hirst. From Werbyn et al.: Br. J. Ophthalmol. 65:403, 1981.)

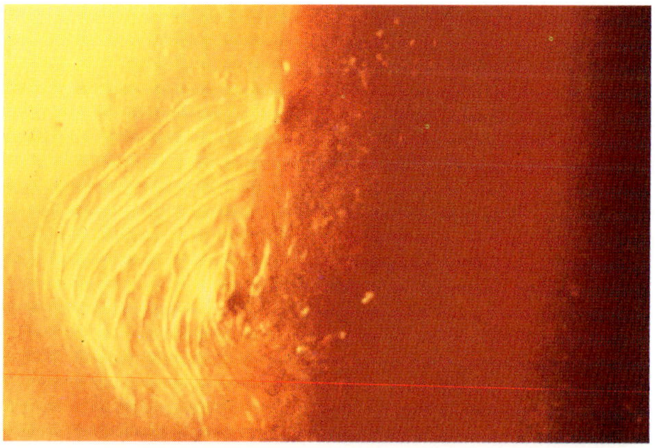

Epithelial basement membrane dystrophy.

Figure 1–6. Multiple "dots" are seen with retroillumination. (Courtesy of Dr. Lawrence Hirst. From Werbyn et al.: Br. J. Ophthalmol. 65:403, 1981.)

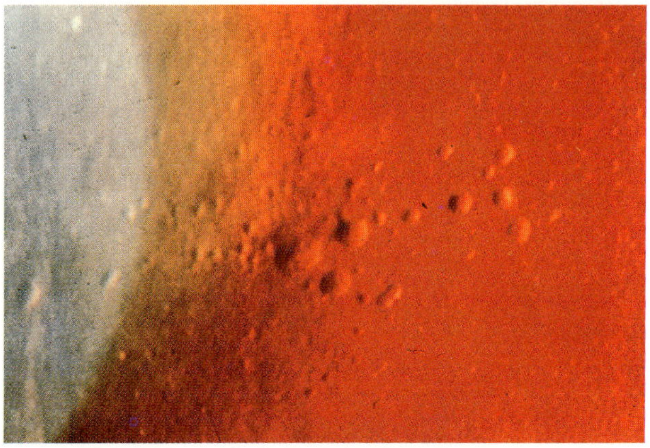

Epithelial basement membrane dystrophy.

Figure 1–7. Characteristic, irregular tear film is demonstrated in the dystrophic area with fluorescein dye and cobalt blue filter.

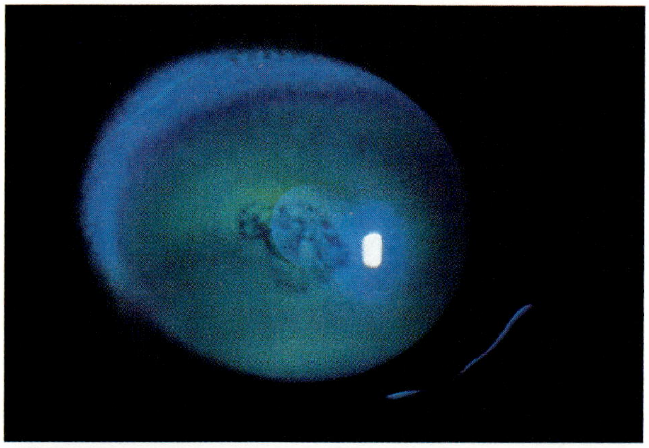

Reis-Buckler dystrophy.

Figure 1–8. Diffuse, reticular subepithelial corneal opacification at the level of Bowman's membrane is present throughout the entire cornea. The corneal surface is rough and irregular.

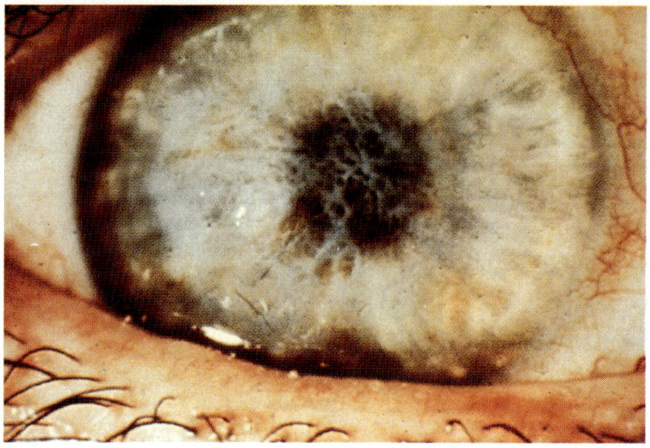

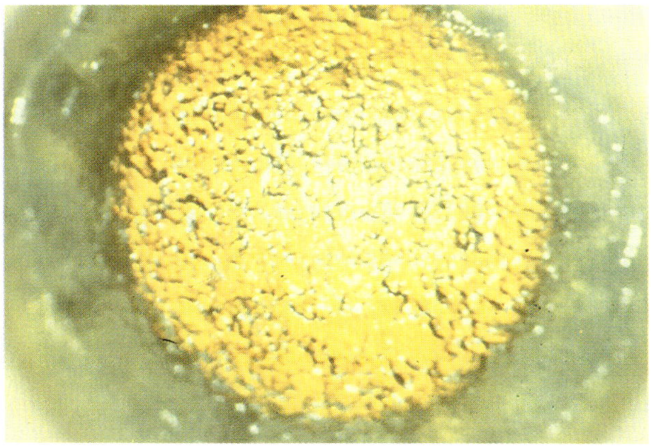

Reis-Buckler dystrophy.

Figure 1–9. After epithelial removal, marked irregularity of Bowman's membrane is demonstrated with retroillumination.

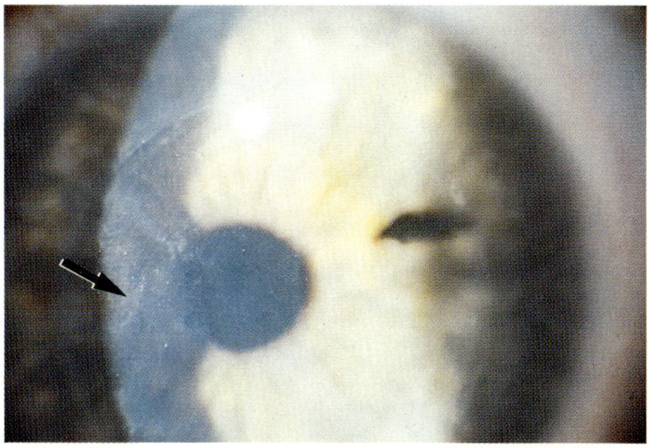

Reis-Buckler dystrophy.

Figure 1–10. Fine, subepithelial refractile lines are seen temporally (arrow) as the first evidence of recurrence in this three-year-old corneal transplant.

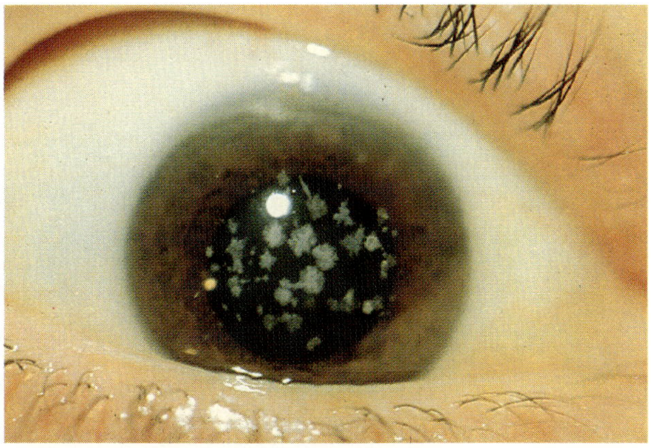

Granular dystrophy.

Figure 1–11. Opacities resembling "bread crumbs" are present axially. The opacities extend from the anterior cornea to the mid-stroma. Uninvolved areas are crystal clear.

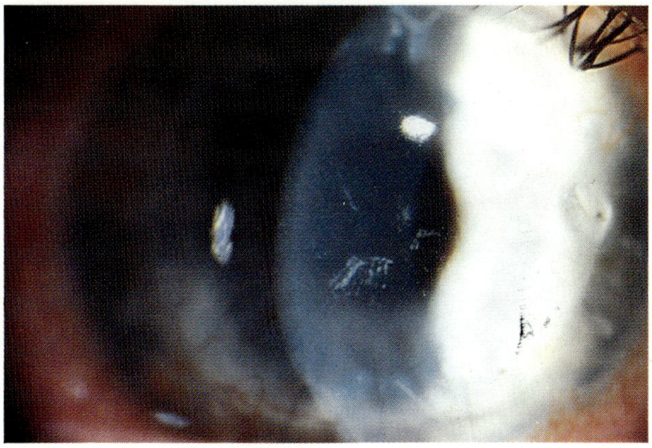

Granular dystrophy.

Figure 1–12. Recurrence of granular dystrophy in this corneal transplant is seen as fine, subepithelial refractile lines in the axial portion of the graft. The recurrent dystrophy in this graft is indistinguishable from the recurrent Reis-Buckler dystrophy seen in Figure 1–10.

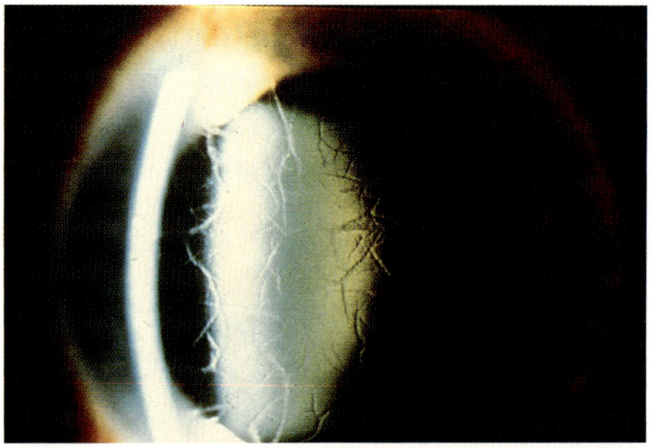

Lattice dystrophy.

Figure 1–13. Refractile lines in a lattice pattern are present from limbus to limbus. The cornea remains clear in uninvolved areas.

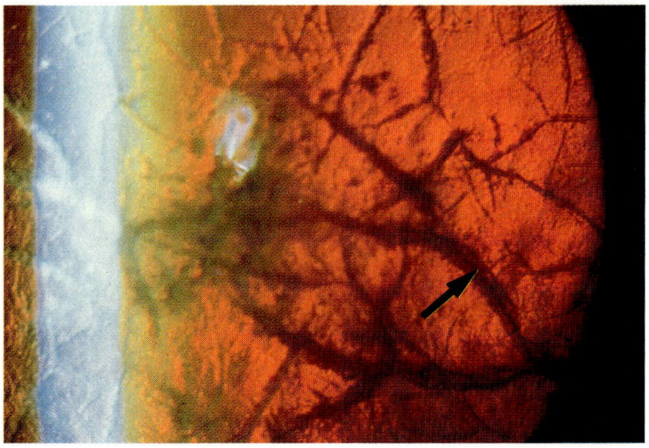

Lattice dystrophy.

Figure 1–14. In retroillumination, several of the lattice lines are thicker and have a "ropy" appearance (arrow). There is a dense central grayish opacity that has resulted in decreased visual acuity. This is a more advanced case than in Figure 1–13.

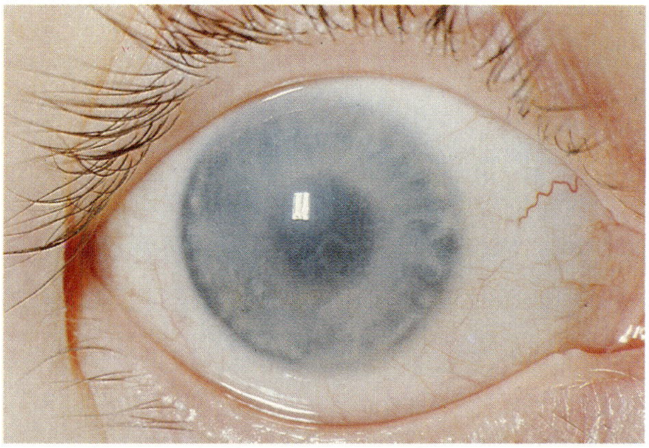

Macular dystrophy.

Figure 1–15. Diffuse stromal opacification gives a "ground glass" appearance of the entire cornea. Centrally there are diffuse, grayish-white opacities with indistinct edges.

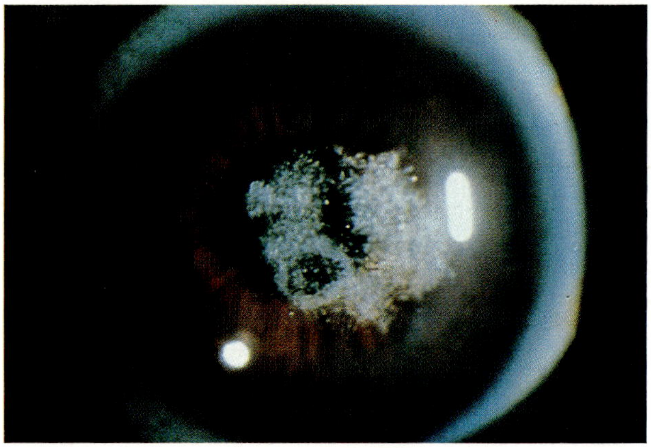

Central crystalline dystrophy (Schnyder's dystrophy).

Figure 1–16. Fine, needle-shaped, polychromatic crystals form an annular opacity with a clear center (donut pattern).

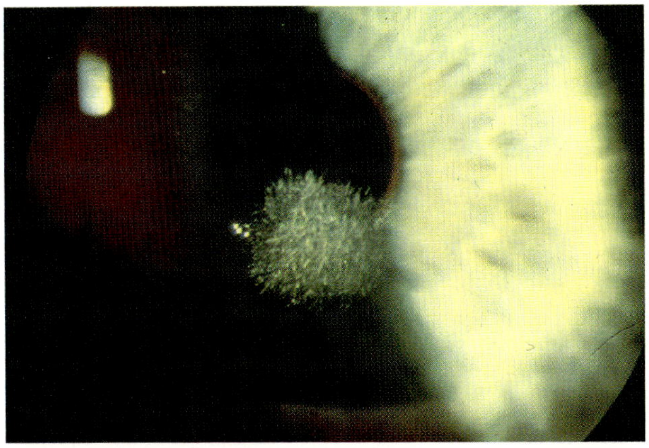

Central crystalline dystrophy.

Figure 1–17. In a pattern less commonly seen than that in Figure 1–16, the crystals form a discoid lesion with an ill-defined edge.

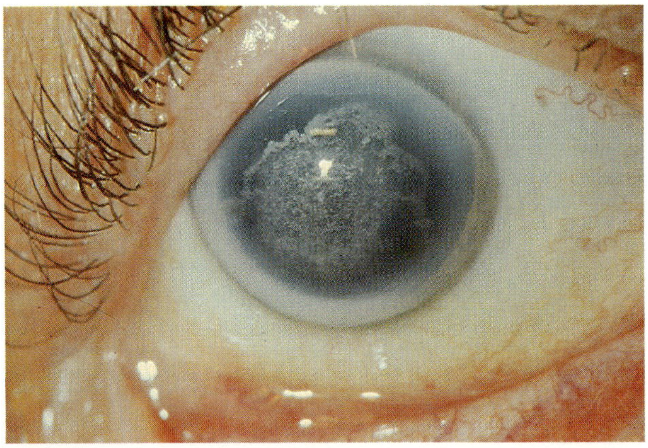

Central crystalline dystrophy.

Figure 1–18. Similar pattern to that seen in Figure 1–17, but with more extensive involvement of the central cornea. Note the associated arcus senilis.

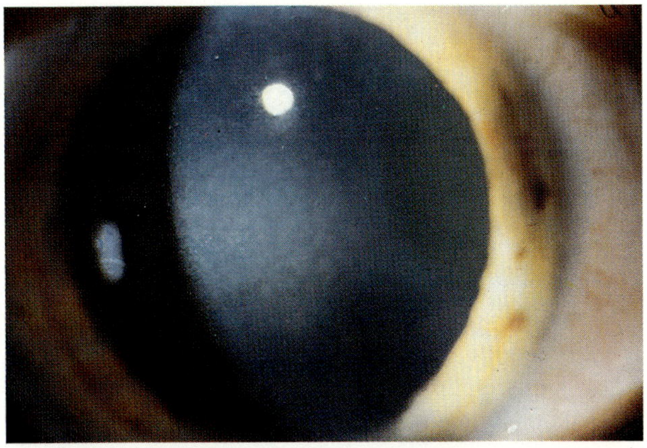

Central cloudy dystrophy (Francois' dystrophy).

Figure 1–19. Opacification is seen in the deep (posterior third), central cornea. The lesion consists of multiple small, fuzzy, marginated gray areas in a polygonal pattern separated by clear, cracklike zones.

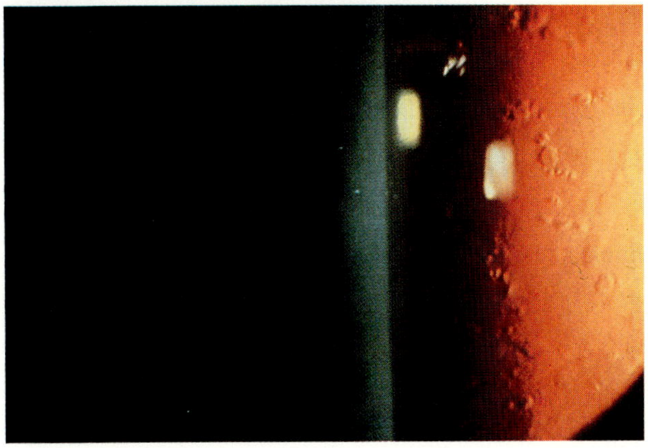

Posterior polymorphous dystrophy.

Figure 1–20. Multiple small vesicles surrounded by diffuse gray halos at the level of, or just anterior to, Descemet's membrane are highlighted by retroillumination. Thickened areas of Descemet's membrane can be seen temporally.

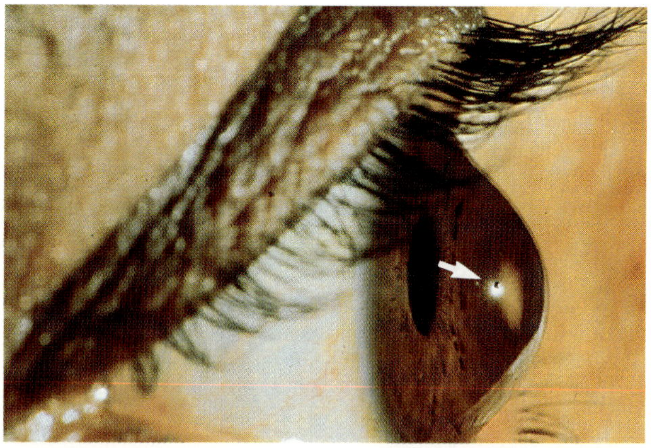

Keratoconus.

Figure 1–21. Lateral view of marked central corneal ectasia. Axial stromal scarring is present (arrow).

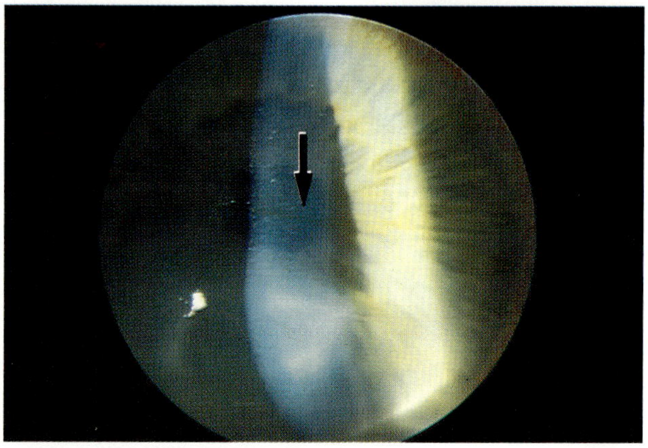

Keratoconus.

Figure 1–22. Anterior stromal scarring is present inferior to the visual axis. Superiorly an iron pigment ring (Fleischer ring) is present (arrow).

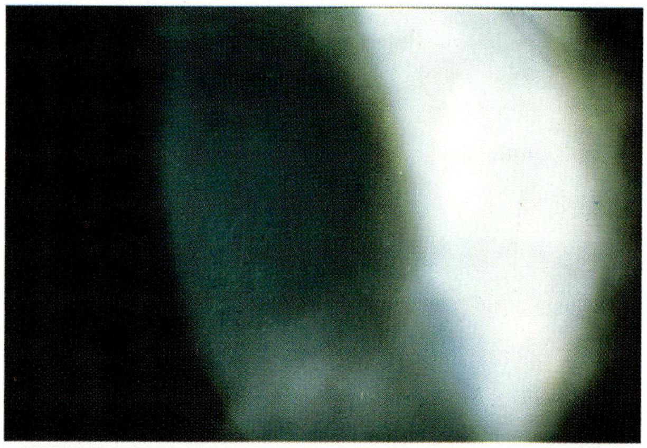

Keratoconus.

Figure 1–23. Vertical striae (Vogt's lines) are present in the deep corneal stroma.

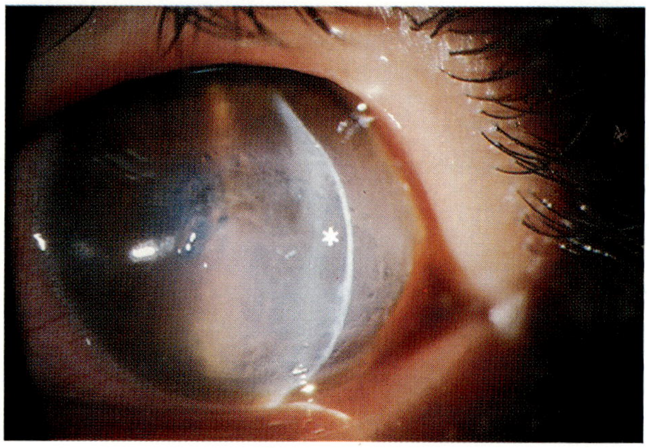

Keratoconus.

Figure 1–24. Rupture of Descemet's membrane with resultant corneal stromal edema (hydrops) is present. An intrastromal water cleft can be seen (asterisk).

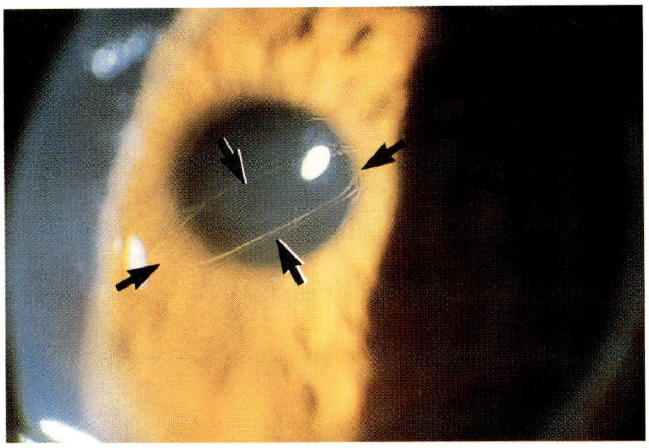

Keratoconus.

Figure 1–25. A "fish mouth" opening in Descemet's membrane remains following resolution of corneal hydrops (arrows).

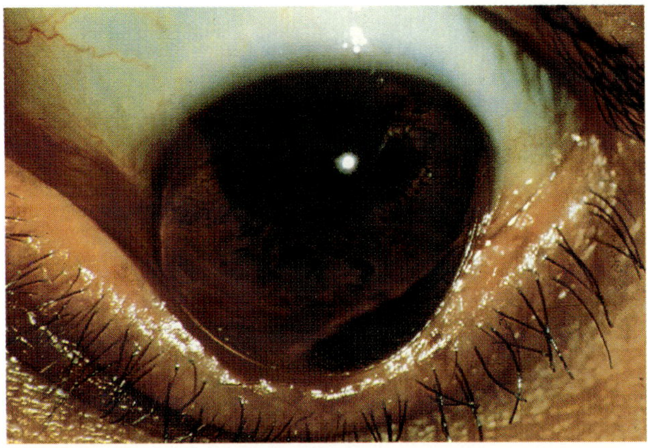

Keratoglobus.

Figure 1–26. Complete ectasia of the cornea is present. On downgaze a characteristic concave distortion of the lower lid (Munson's sign) is demonstrated.

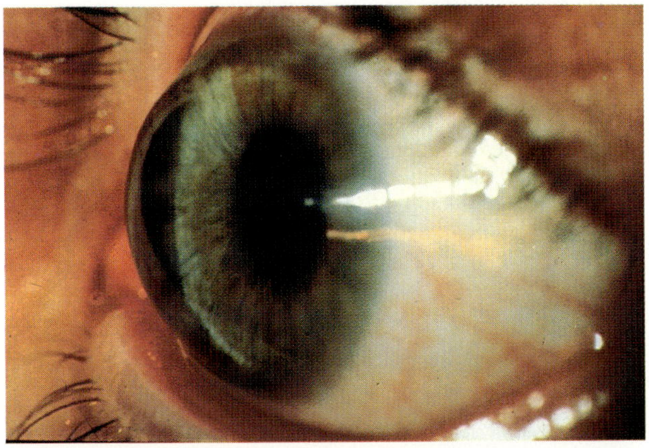

Keratoglobus.

Figure 1–27. Lateral view of cornea with complete ectasia.

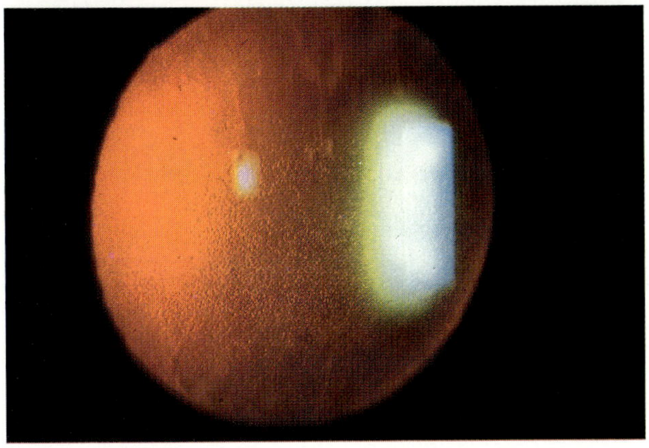

Fuchs' dystrophy.

Figure 1–28. Extensive endothelial guttata are demonstrated by retroillumination.

Fuchs' dystrophy.

Figure 1–29. Guttata and characteristic endothelial pigment dusting are seen by slit lamp biomicroscopy.

Fuchs' dystrophy.

Figure 1–30. Guttata, thickening of Descemet's membrane with some loss of clarity, and stromal edema are present in this moderately advanced case.

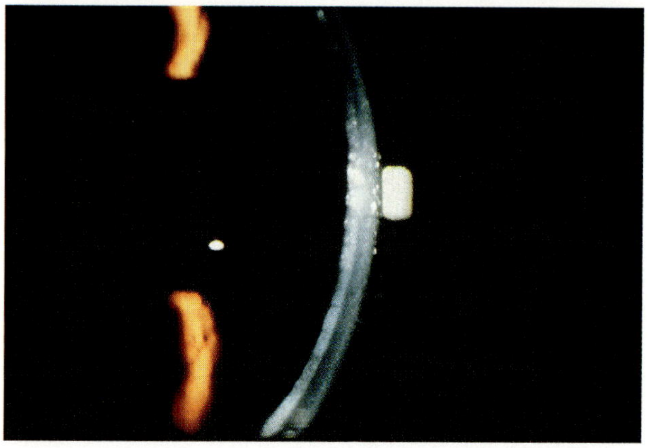

Fuchs' dystrophy.

Figure 1–31. Stromal edema and epithelial microcystic edema are present. The microcystic edema is well highlighted by fluorescein staining and examination with a cobalt blue filter.

Fuchs' dystrophy.

Figure 1–32. Inflammation from ruptured epithelial bullae has resulted in sterile hypopyon.

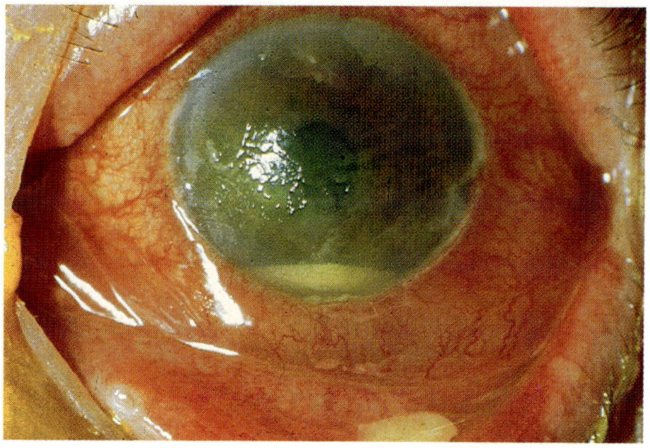

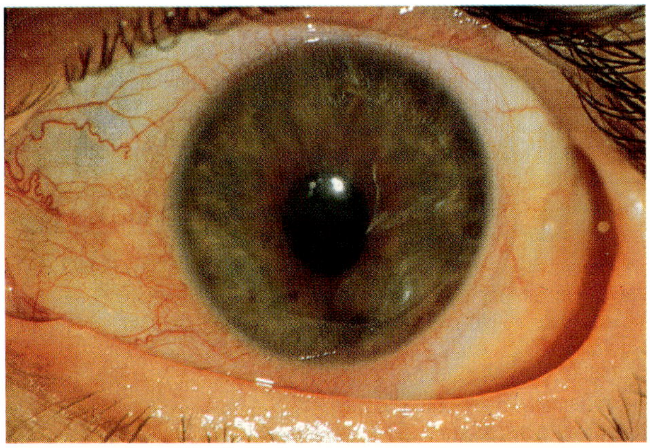

Iridocorneal endothelial syndrome (Chandler's syndrome).

Figure 1–33. Mild corneal stromal edema is present. The presence of peripheral anterior synechia at 6:00 is suggested by the slight distortion of the pupil in that meridian.

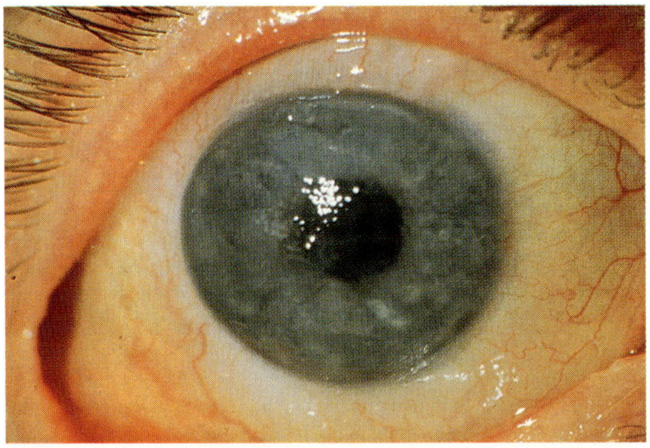

Iridocorneal endothelial syndrome (Chandler's syndrome).

Figure 1–34. Stromal and epithelial edema are present. There are no abnormalities of the pupil or iris.

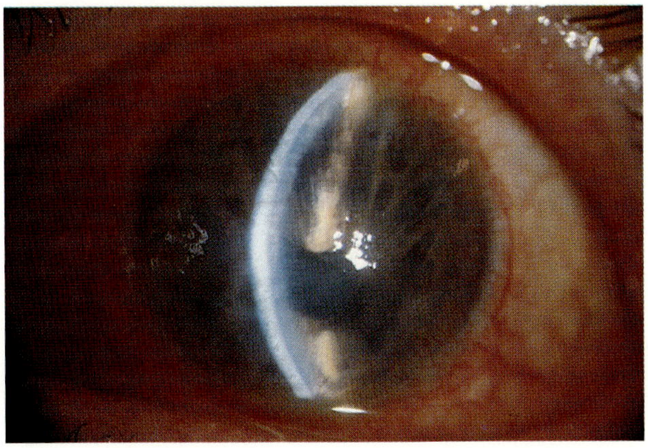

Iridocorneal endothelial syndrome (essential iris atrophy).

Figure 1–35. Corneal stromal and epithelial edema are present along with multiple full-thickness iris holes. The pupil is dragged inferiorly by peripheral anterior synechia.

2

Corneal Degenerations

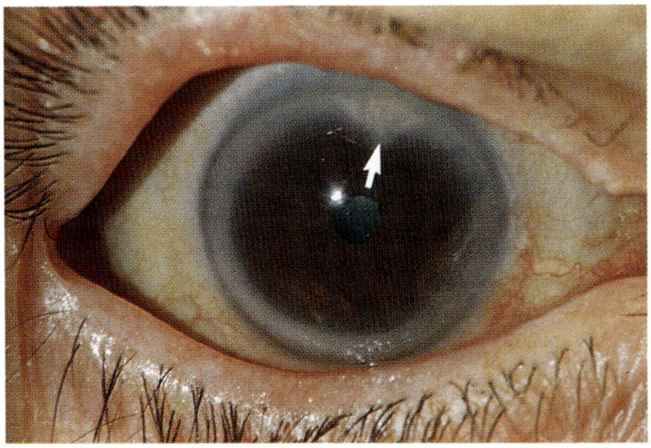

Arcus senilis.

Figure 2–1. A yellowish-white deposition of lipid, not associated with vascularization, is present in a 360° concentric pattern separated from the corneal limbus by a lucid interval. Superiorly (arrow) a small area of additional lipid deposition is present in association with superior limbic vasculature.

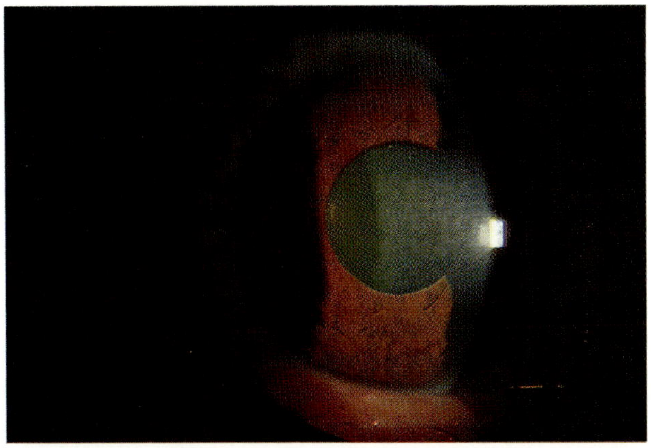

Mosaic (crocodile) shagreen of Vogt.

Figure 2–2. Grayish-white polygonal opacities separated by clear spaces are seen in the anterior, central cornea.

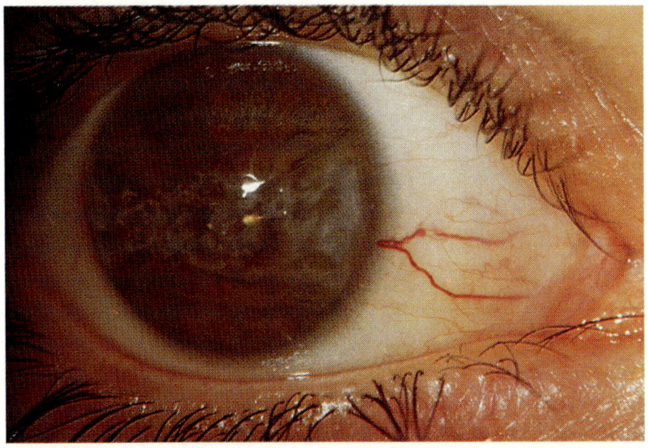

Band keratopathy.

Figure 2–3. Calcific deposits are deposited at the level of Bowman's membrane in the interpalpebral fissure. Note the clear zone present at the limbus, and numerous holes in the band, representing sites of penetration of corneal nerves through Bowman's membrane.

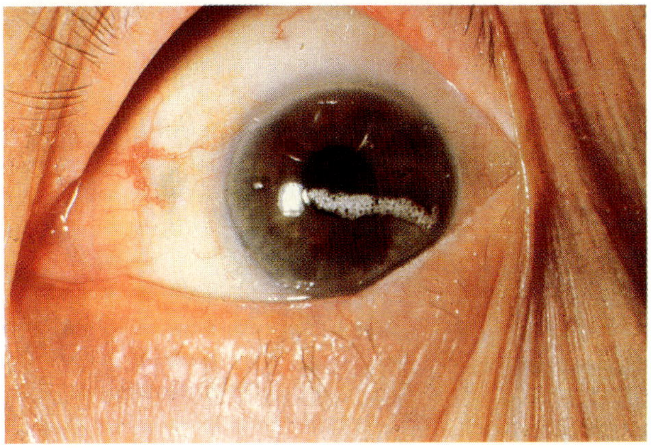

Band keratopathy.

Figure 2–4. Calcium deposition in this cornea is limited to the most exposed portion of the interpalpebral zone.

Lipid keratopathy.

Figure 2–5. A dense, white deposition of lipid with feathery edges has occurred in association with superior limbic pannus (arrow). This is much more advanced than that seen in Figure 2–1. Note that this eye has previously undergone an intracapsular cataract extraction and subsequent secondary implantation of an anterior chamber IOL.

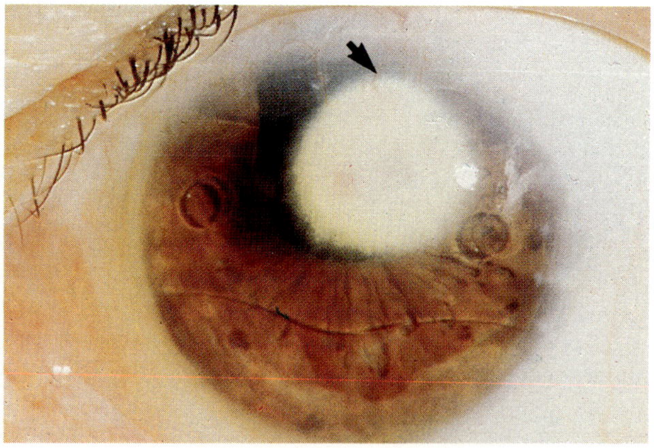

Primary amyloidosis.

Figure 2–6. Classic appearance of a raised, gelatinous mass with a "mulberry" surface due to primary deposition of amyloid. The peripheral cornea is clear and there is no vascularization.

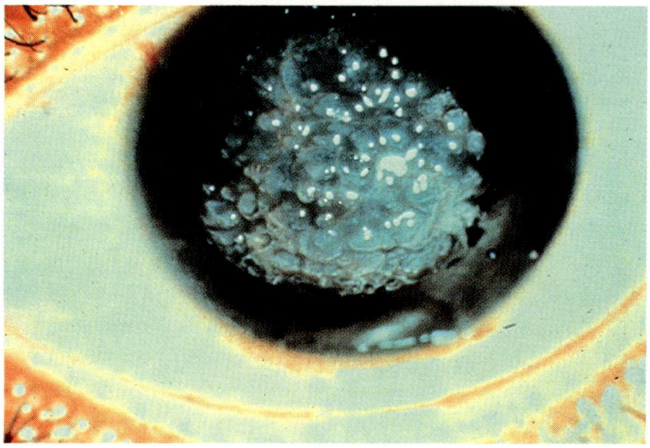

Secondary amyloidosis.

Figure 2–7. Secondary deposition of amyloid (asterisk) has occurred following the development of aphakic bullous keratopathy. In contrast to the appearance of Figure 2–6, peripheral vascularization (arrow) is associated with secondary amyloidosis.

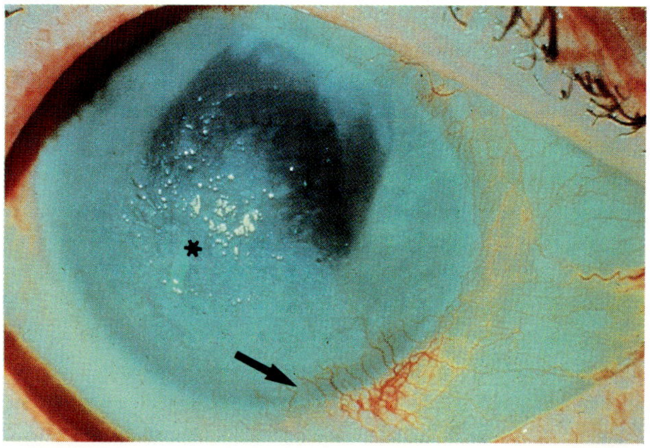

Vortex keratopathy secondary to amiodarone.

Figure 2–8. Whirllike opacification of the epithelium in a vortex pattern is seen in this patient on amiodarone therapy.

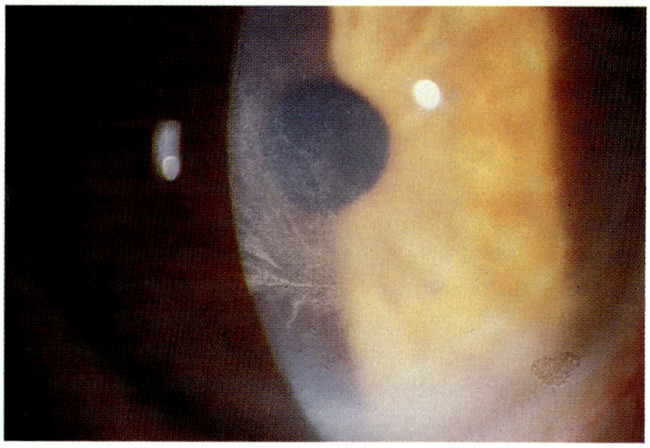

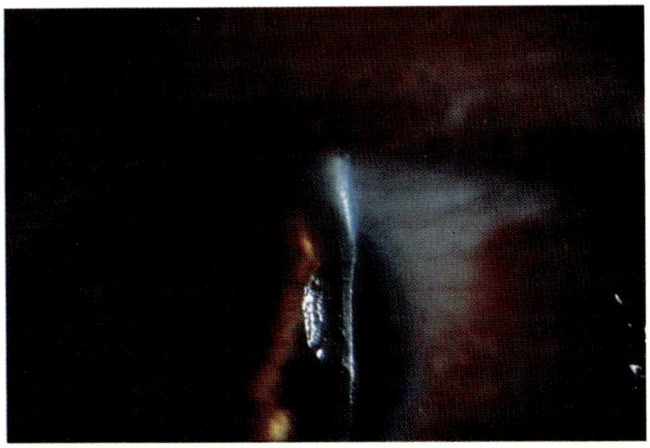

Dellen.

Figure 2–9. A depression in the peripheral cornea is associated with the limbal swelling seen following strabismus surgery. There is no epithelial defect.

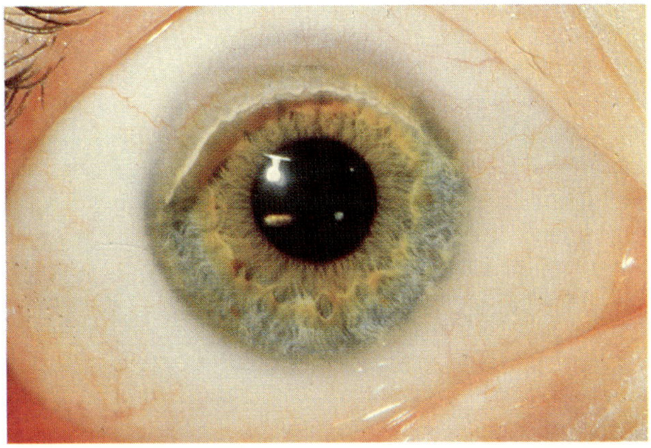

Terrien's marginal degeneration.

Figure 2–10. A superior limbic gutter extends circumferentially from 9:00 to 2:00 (classic distribution). The gutter is vascularized throughout, and there is lipid deposition at the anterior edge of the gutter. The epithelium is intact, and the eye is uninflamed.

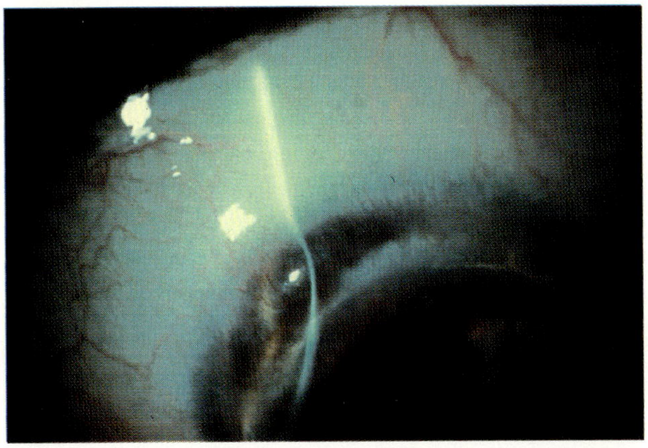

Terrien's marginal degeneration.

Figure 2–11. On down gaze, a slit beam demonstrates extreme thinning, vascularization, and lipid deposition.

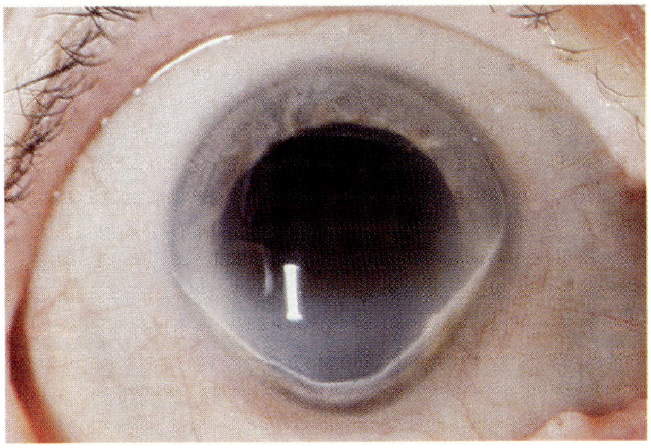

Terrien's marginal degeneration.

Figure 2–12. Atypical distribution of peripheral marginal thinning circumferentially along the inferior limbus. Diagnosis is made on the basis of previous recurrent episodes of ocular inflammation, as well as the presence of vascularization in the gutter and lipid deposition at the leading edge. Astigmatic error of 18 diopters is present.

Pellucid degeneration.

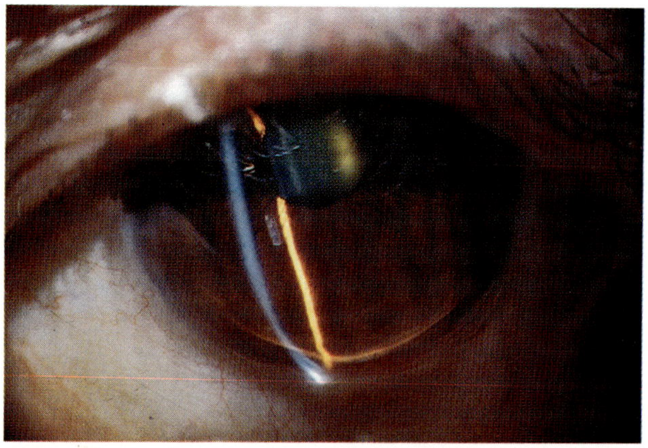

Figure 2–13. Thinning of the inferior limbus is seen in the absence of vascularization or lipid deposition, in contrast to Figure 2–12.

Salzmann's nodular degeneration.

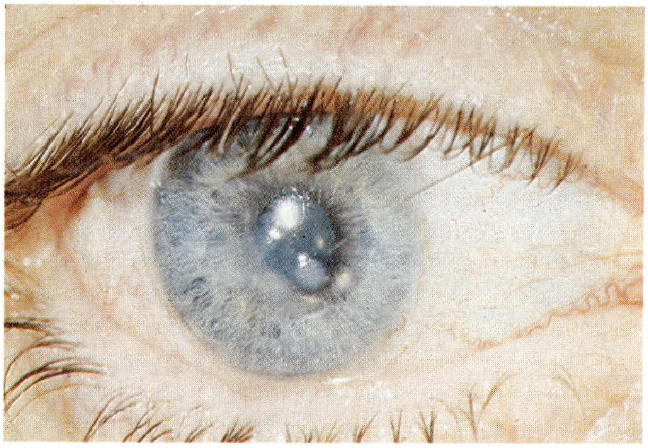

Figure 2–14. Three bluish-gray, elevated nodules are present in the central corneal epithelium in this mild case. The remainder of the cornea is clear.

Salzmann's nodular degeneration.

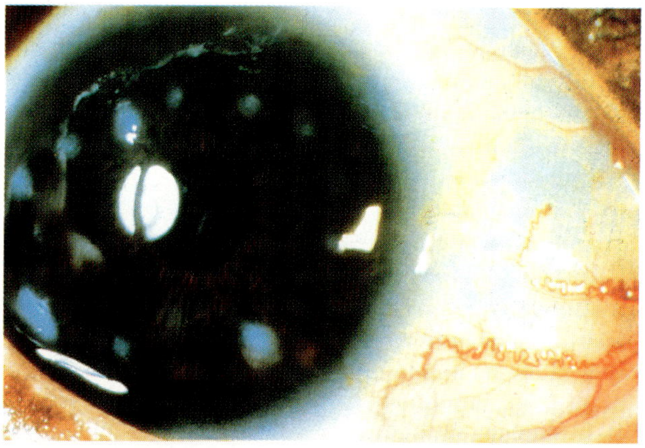

Figure 2–15. Multiple bluish-gray, elevated nodules are present in the classic concentric, para-axial distribution with sparing of the remainder of the cornea.

Salzmann's nodular degeneration.

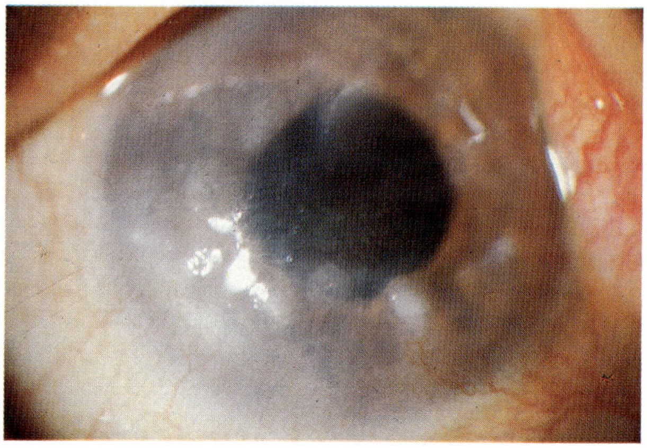

Figure 2–16. In the same eye shown in Figure 2–15 (ten years later), atypical peripheral vascularization and loss of clarity between the nodules has occurred.

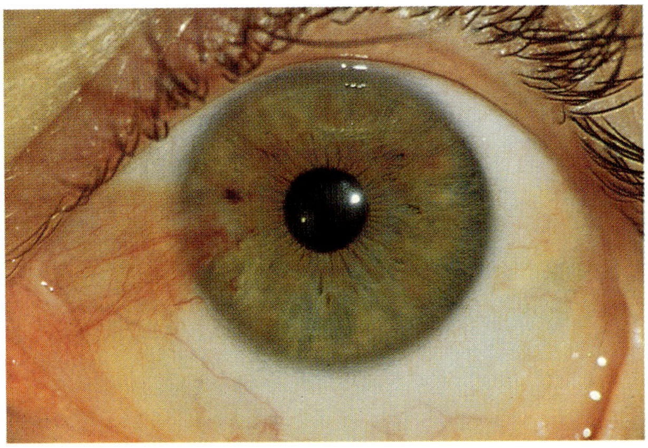

Pterygium.

Figure 2–17. Thickened, inflamed vascular tissue has extended 1 mm onto the corneal limbus in this early pterygium.

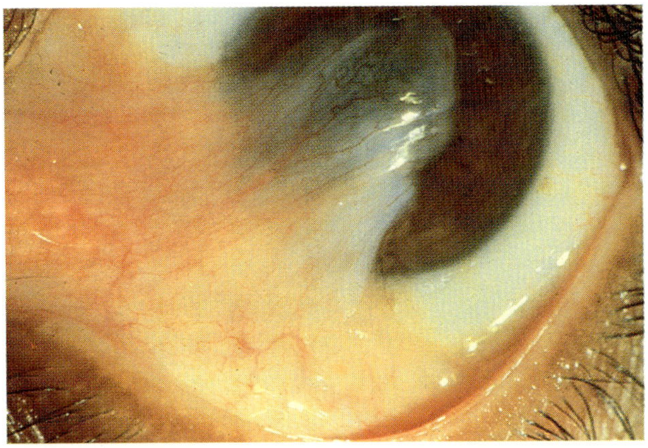

Pterygium.

Figure 2–18. In this patient of Caribbean origin, a neglected pterygium has extended across the visual axis.

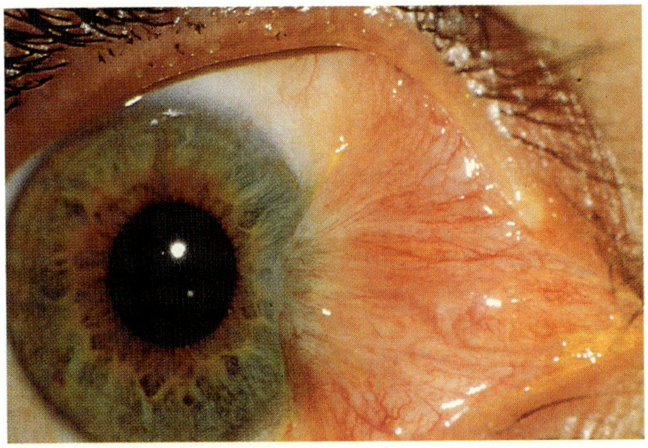

Recurrent pterygium.

Figure 2–19. Following primary pterygium resection, an intensely inflamed recurrent pterygium involving the entire medial aspect of the globe, with restriction of adduction, has occurred.

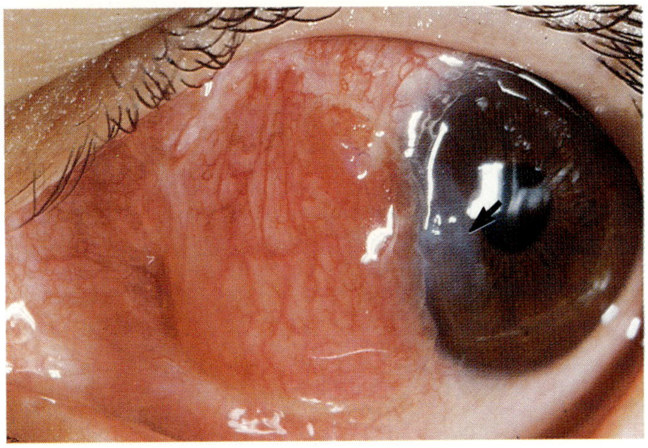

Recurrent pterygium, s/p excision and transplantation of free conjunctival graft.

Figure 2–20. One week following excision of pterygium, residual scarring of the corneal bed is seen (arrow). The free conjunctival graft is edematous and well vascularized (normal appearance).

3

Infections

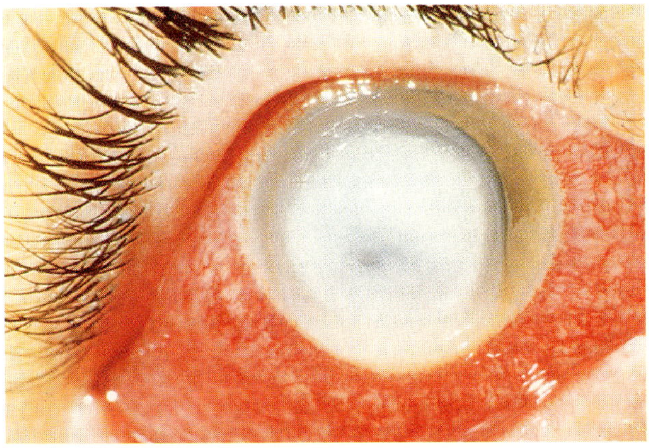

Bacterial keratitis (*Pseudomonas aeruginosa*, acute).

Figure 3–1. Full-thickness, necrotic, gray-white infiltrate with an 80 per cent epithelial defect and hypopyon in extended soft contact lens wearer.

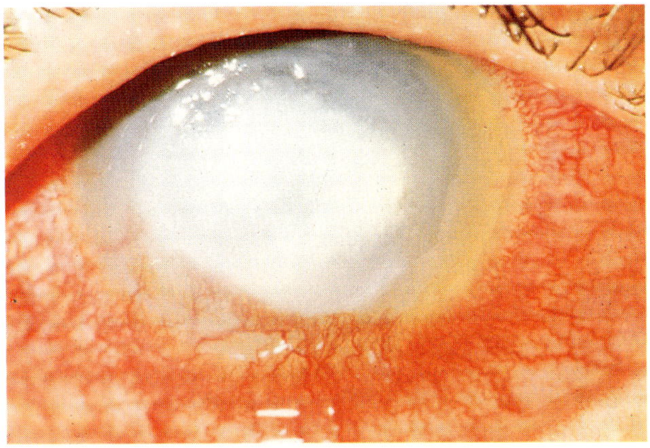

Bacterial keratitis (*Pseudomonas aeruginosa*, resolving).

Figure 3–2. One month after presentation, the infiltrate is less extensive, the size of the epithelial defect is reduced, and no perforation has occurred. Peripheral vascularization is prominent inferotemporally.

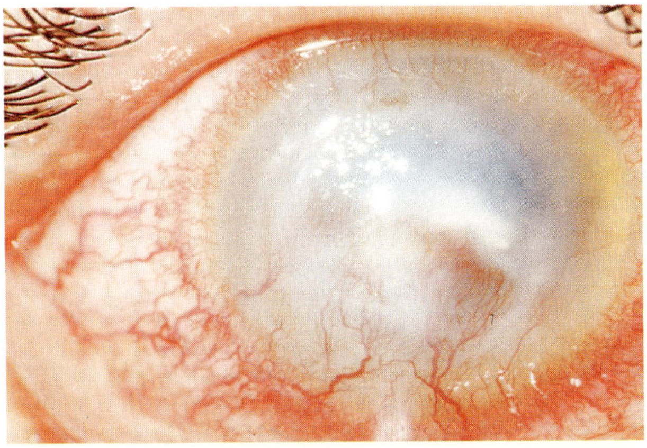

Bacterial keratitis (*Pseudomonas aeruginosa*, resolving).

Figure 3–3. Virtual resolution of corneal infiltrate after two months of antimicrobial therapy. Severe corneal vascularization and scar formation have resulted.

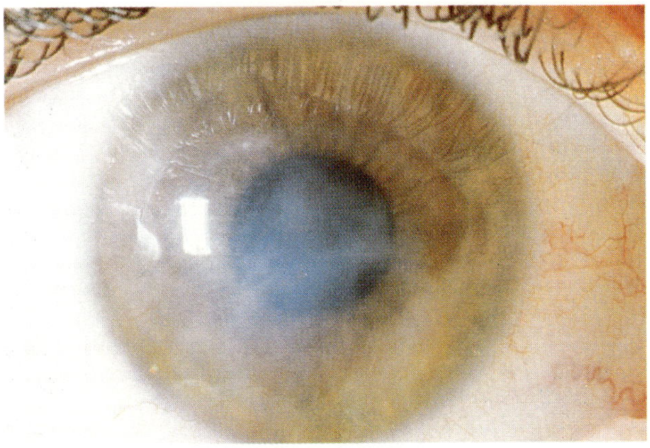

Bacterial keratitis (*Pseudomonas aeruginosa*, resolved).

Figure 3–4. After 18 months, significant regression of the vascularization has occurred, but some corneal scarring persists.

Bacterial keratitis (*Proteus vulgaris,* acute).

Figure 3–5. Eight months following penetrating keratoplasty, and two days following removal of an interrupted suture, a dense yellow-white infiltrate developed at the graft-host junction with extension to the limbus. Partial dehiscence of the wound with shallowing of the anterior chamber is present.

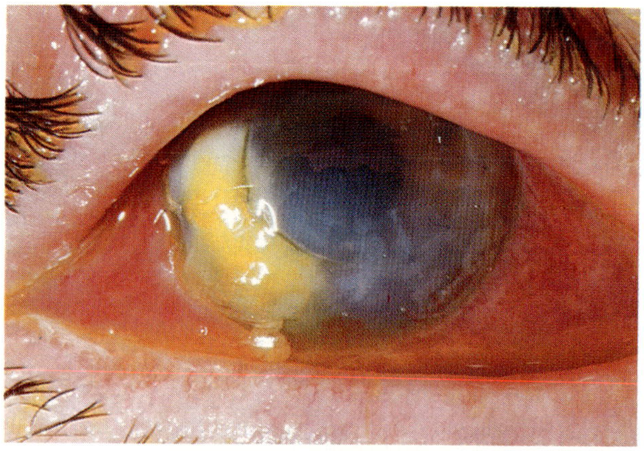

Bacterial keratitis (*Proteus vulgaris,* resolving).

Figure 3–6. One week later, peripheral clearing of the infiltrate has begun. Anterior bulging of the graft still persists, but the anterior chamber has reformed.

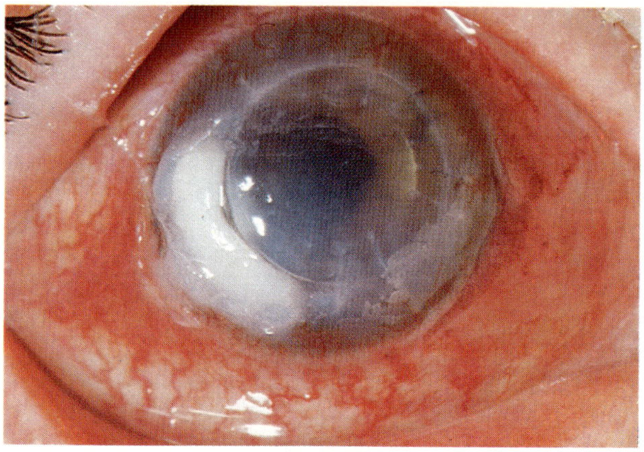

Bacterial keratitis (*Proteus vulgaris,* resolving).

Figure 3–7. Six weeks after presentation, the infiltrate has virtually resolved, peripheral vascularization has begun, and scarring at the graft-host junction has resulted in reestablishment of a secure wound.

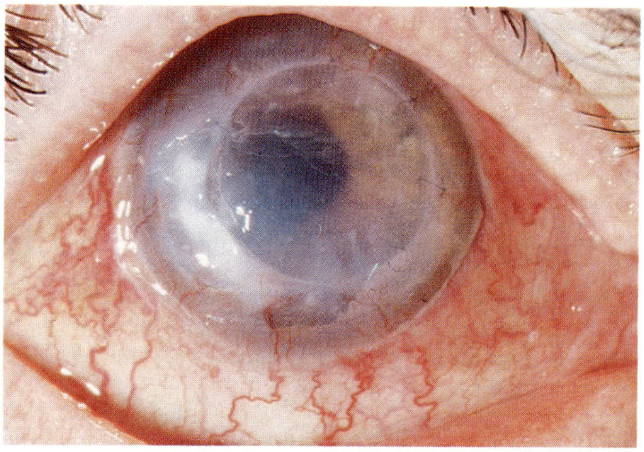

Bacterial keratitis (*Proteus vulgaris,* resolved).

Figure 3–8. Three months later, the infiltrate has resolved and the wound is secure, but the graft has become irreversibly edematous.

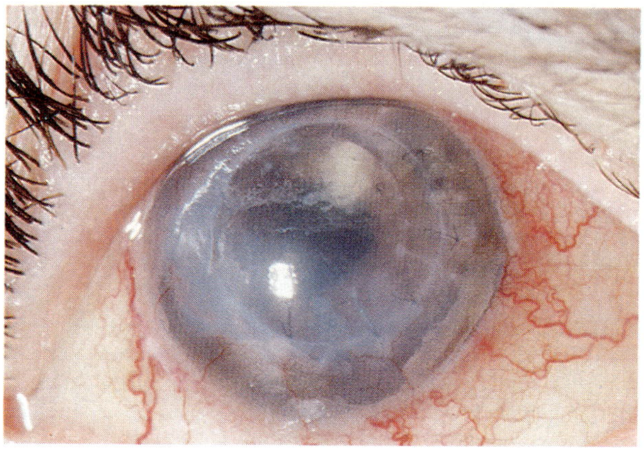

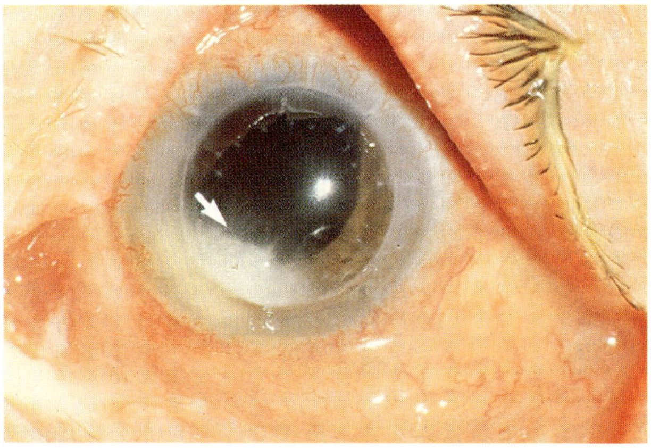

Bacterial keratitis (*Streptococcus viridans*).

Figure 3–9. Characteristic arborizing, crystallike infiltrates in the deep corneal stroma (arrow) are seen due to infection with *Streptococcus viridans*.

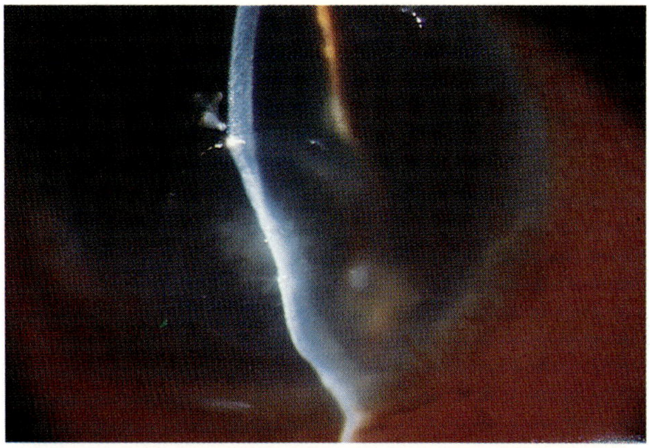

Bacterial keratitis (*Staphylococcus aureus*).

Figure 3–10. A persistent epithelial defect, in a patient with Kearne-Sayre syndrome, has become secondarily infected with *Staphylococcus aureus*. A dense, well-circumscribed stromal infiltrate, associated with stromal loss, is present in the center of the epithelial defect.

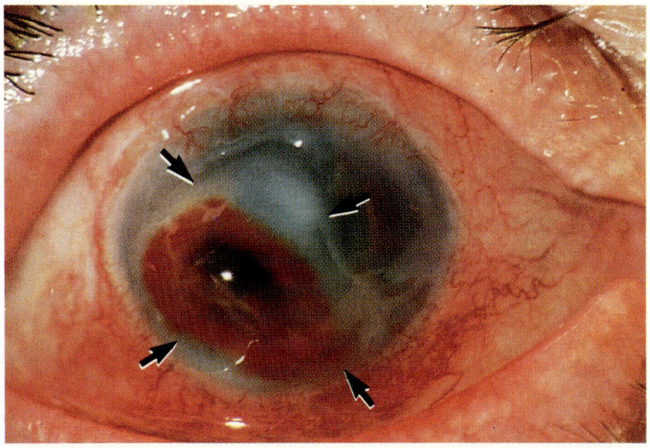

Bacterial keratitis (*Streptococcus pneumoniae*).

Figure 3–11. Soft contact lens wearer who presented with a large epithelial defect (outlined by arrows), extensive stromal infiltrate, and perforated descemetocele with iris prolapse. Significant vascular pannus is present superiorly.

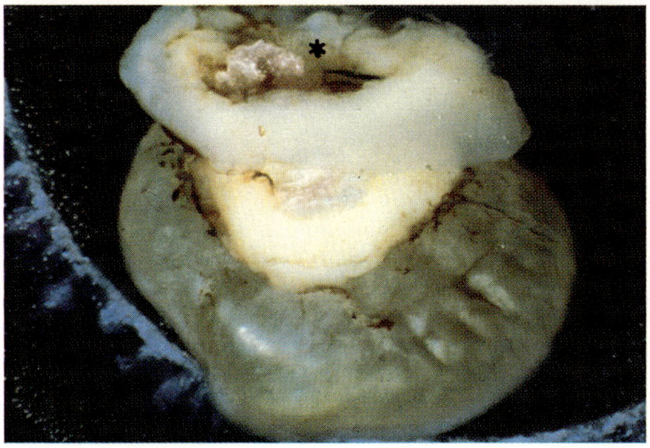

Bacterial keratitis (*Pseudomonas aeruginosa*).

Figure 3–12. "En bloc" surgical specimen consisting of cornea, anterior chamber organized fibrin, and lens from one-eyed patient with advanced *Pseudomonas aeruginosa* infection involving 80 per cent of his cornea with a 7 mm perforation (asterisk).

Fungal keratitis.

Figure 3–13. Fungal contamination of an aphakic soft contact lens following penetrating keratoplasty has not yet involved the cornea.

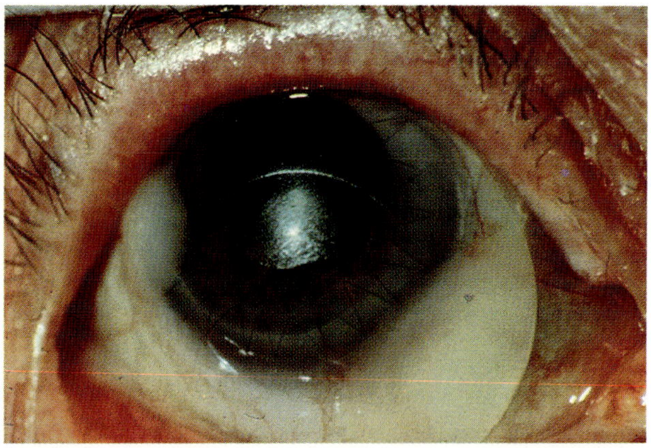

Fungal keratitis.

Figure 3–14. Multiple small "satellite" infiltrates are seen in association with two small epithelial defects. Unlike the corneas shown in Figures 3–16 to 3–18, the initial presentation in this case was not florid.

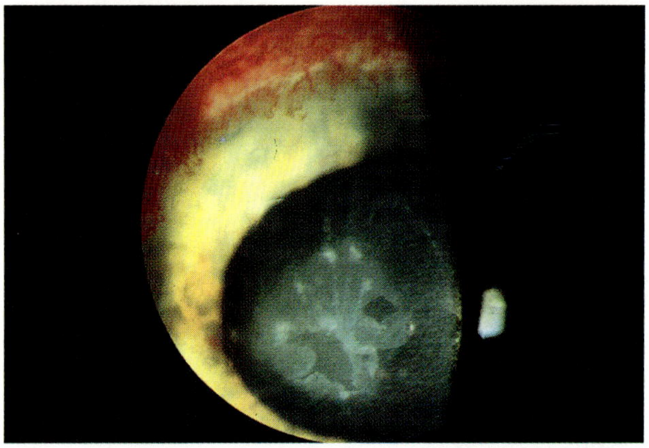

Fungal keratitis (*Candida albicans*).

Figure 3–15. A small, deep stromal infiltrate with feathery edges adjacent to a corneal suture grew abundant *Candida albicans* on culture. The epithelial defect was not present until the infiltrate was cultured.

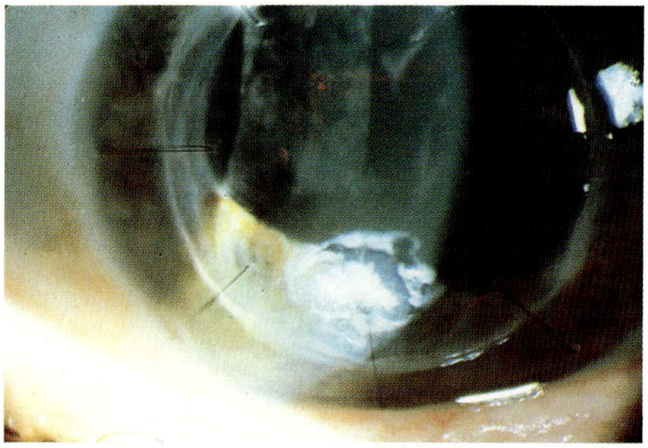

Fungal keratitis (*Fusarium*).

Figure 3–16. Classic appearance of fungal keratitis with dense stromal infiltrate associated with multiple "satellite" lesions and an anterior chamber hypopyon.

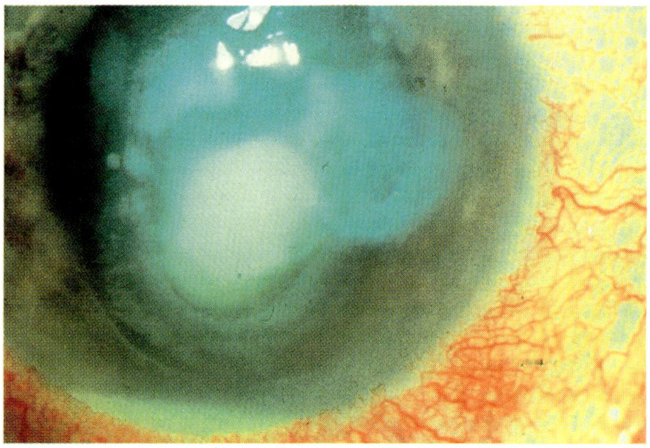

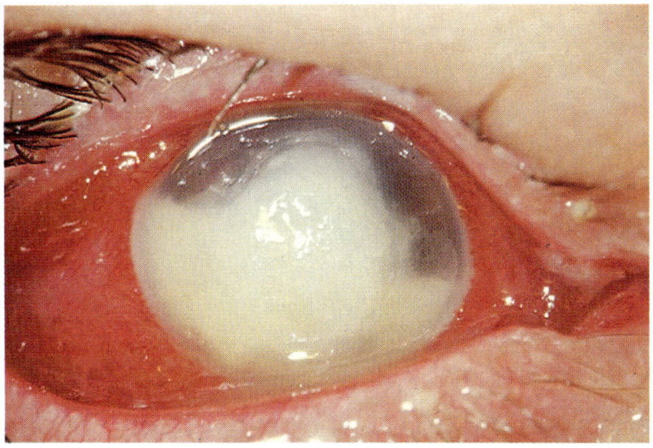

Fungal keratitis (*Fusarium*).

Figure 3–17. Nonclassic yet common presentation of fungal keratitis as an advanced stromal infiltrate without characteristic satellite lesions. Diagnosis was established by corneal biopsy after multiple negative cultures.

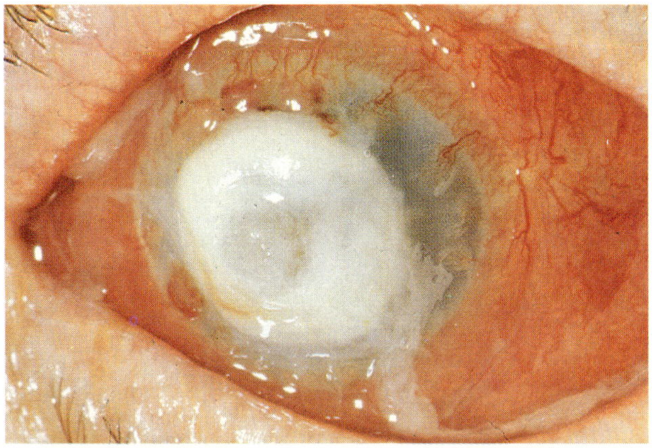

Fungal keratitis (*Penicillium*).

Figure 3–18. Three weeks after application of cyanoacrylate glue for large central descemetocele, removal of glue revealed extensive corneal infiltrate due to *Penicillium* with central perforated descemetocele. Note extensive peripheral vascularization induced by the glue and fungal infection.

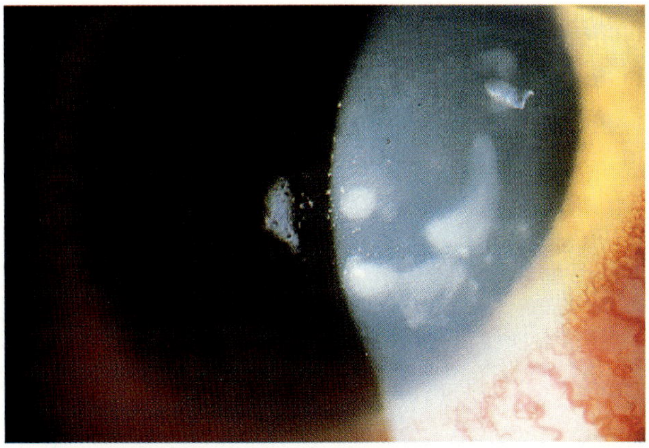

Corneal infiltrate, presumed hypersensitivity.

Figure 3–19. Multiple peripheral corneal infiltrates initially diagnosed as fungal keratitis. After multiple negative cultures for both bacteria and fungi, corneal biopsy was positive only for herpes simplex viral antigens.

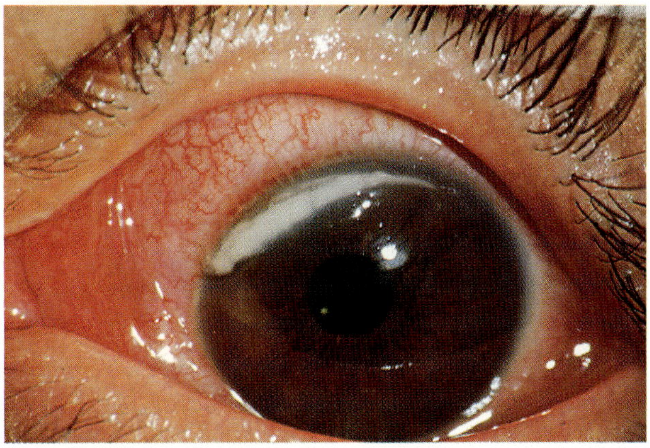

Corneal infiltrate, presumed hypersensitivity.

Figure 3–20. Culture-negative, steroid-responsive peripheral marginal infiltrate with epithelial defect in a patient with no obvious lid disease or rosacea and a negative systemic workup for collagen-vascular disease. Note characteristic "ring" appearance of the infiltrate along the superior corneal limbus, and the small clear zone between the infiltrate and limbus.

Acanthamoeba keratitis.

Figure 3–21. Ring-shaped corneal infiltrate with extensive stromal necrosis in soft contact lens wearer from India. Contralateral eye had almost identical appearance. The diagnosis was established only by examination of the surgical specimen following penetrating keratoplasty.

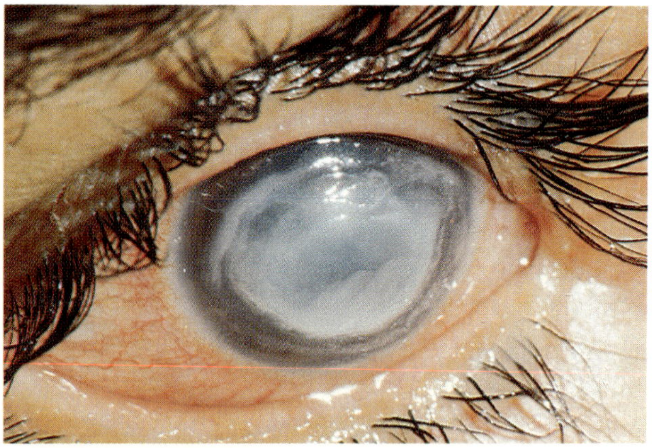

Acanthamoeba keratitis, s/p penetrating keratoplasty.

Figure 3–22. A penetrating keratoplasty seems to have removed all infected portions of the cornea.

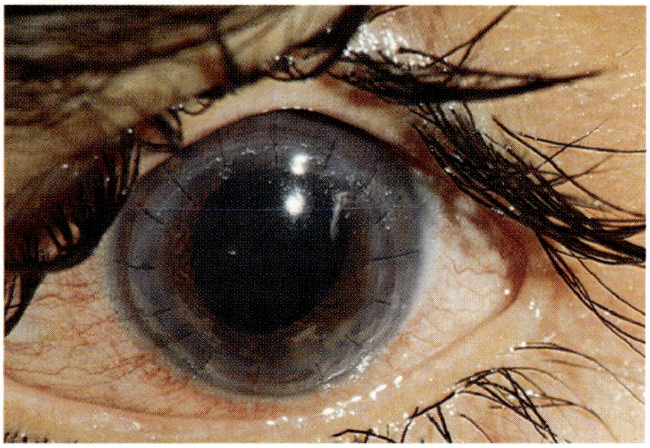

Acanthamoeba keratitis, recurrence in graft.

Figure 3–23. One week following penetrating keratoplasty, a small infiltrate has appeared inferiorly in the graft. The host cornea remains clear.

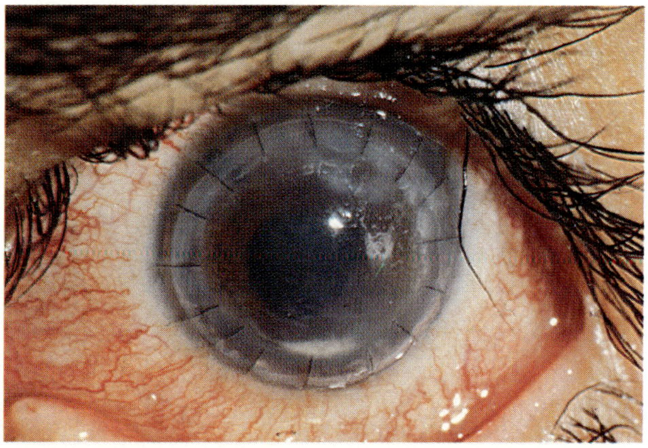

Acanthamoeba keratitis, recurrence in graft.

Figure 3–24. Three days later, the entire graft is involved with a ring-shaped infiltrate that was culture-positive for *Acanthamoeba*.

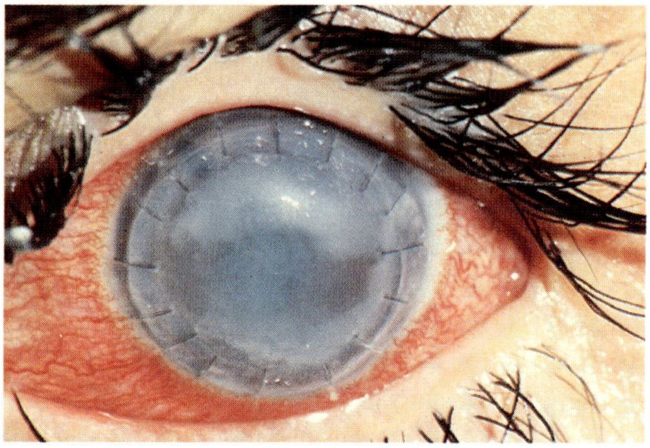

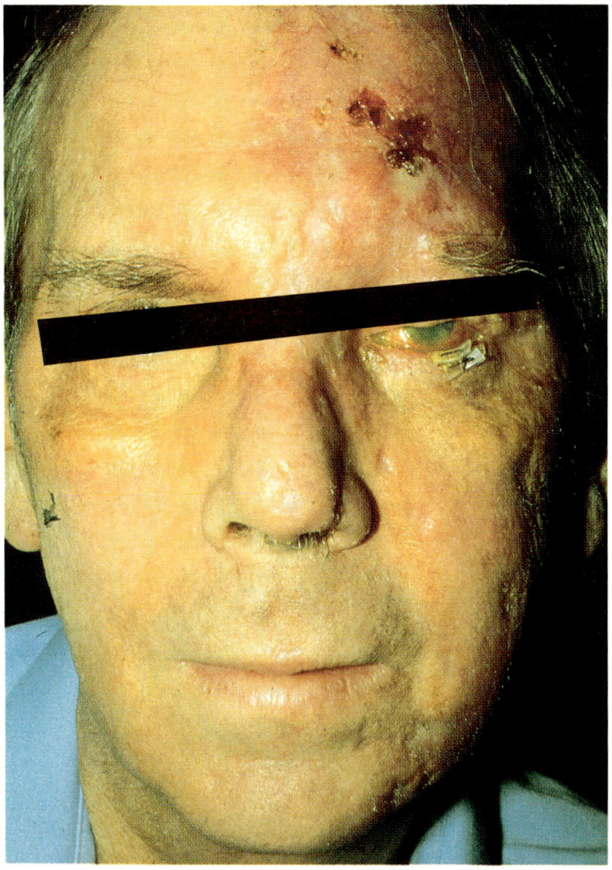

Herpes zoster ophthalmicus.

Figure 3–33. Classic vesicular skin eruptions in the distribution of the first branch of the trigeminal nerve with associated ocular involvement and systemic lymphoma.

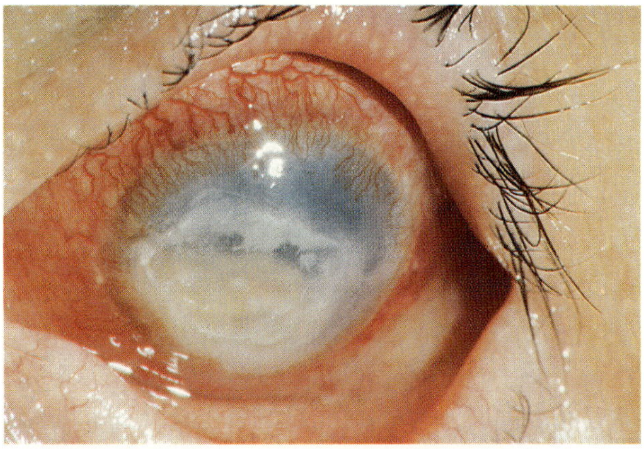

Herpes zoster ophthalmicus.

Figure 3–34. Neurotrophic keratitis due to herpes zoster ophthalmicus with persistent epithelial defect, stromal thinning, and multiple sterile, inflammatory infiltrates.

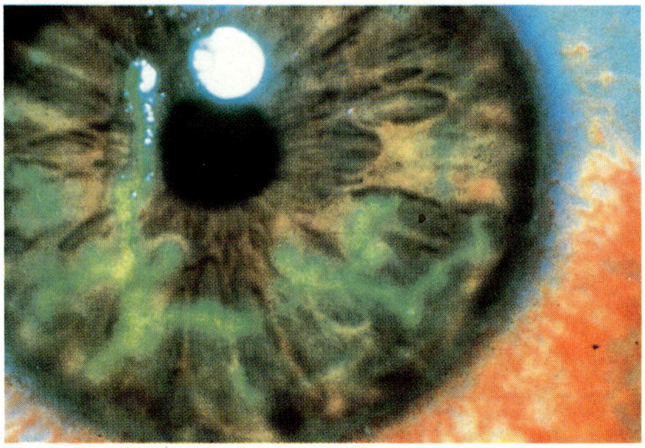

Herpes simplex, epithelial keratitis.

Figure 3–35. Classic fluorescein staining pattern of dendritic, epithelial ulcers due to herpes simplex virus infection. (From Langston, D. (ed.): Ocular Viral Disease International Ophthalmology Clinics, volume 15. Boston, Little, Brown, and Co., 1975.)

Herpes simplex, epithelial keratitis.

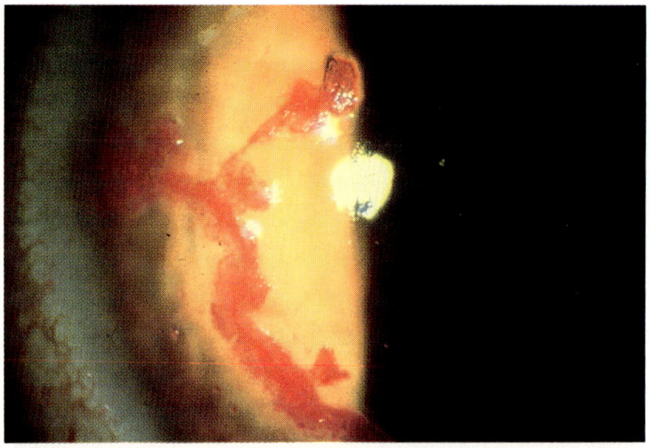

Figure 3–36. Preferential rose bengal staining of intact but actively infected epithelial cells at the leading edge of a dendritic corneal ulcer. Ballooned cells are present along the ulcer margin. This staining pattern is also demonstrated in Figure 3–41.

Herpes simplex, dendrogeographic keratitis.

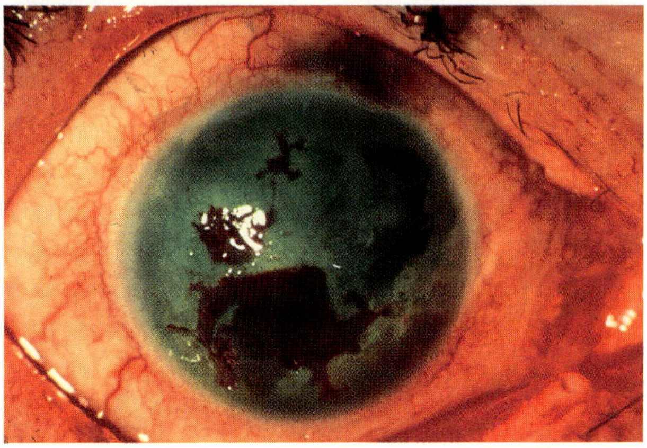

Figure 3–37. Multiple recurrent dendritic, dendrogeographic, and geographic herpes simplex ulcers in cornea with diffuse stromal edema. (From Smolin, G., and Thoft, R. (eds.): The Cornea: Scientific Foundations and Clinical Practice. Boston, Little, Brown, and Co., 1983.)

Herpes simplex, geographic keratitis.

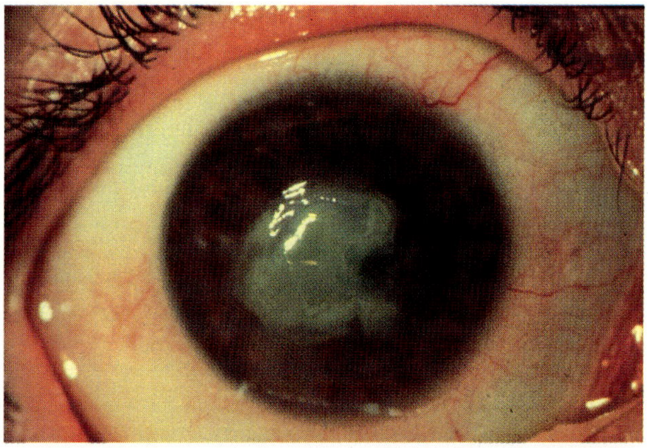

Figure 3–38. Large, ameboid, geographic ulcer in patient on topical corticosteroid therapy for stromal keratitis.

Pseudodendrite.

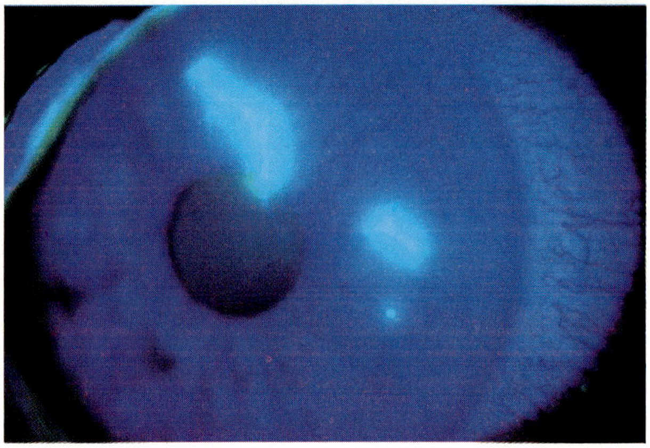

Figure 3–39. Dendritic pattern of epithelial fluorescein staining due to rupture of multiple intraepithelial cysts in cornea with map-dot-fingerprint dystrophy.

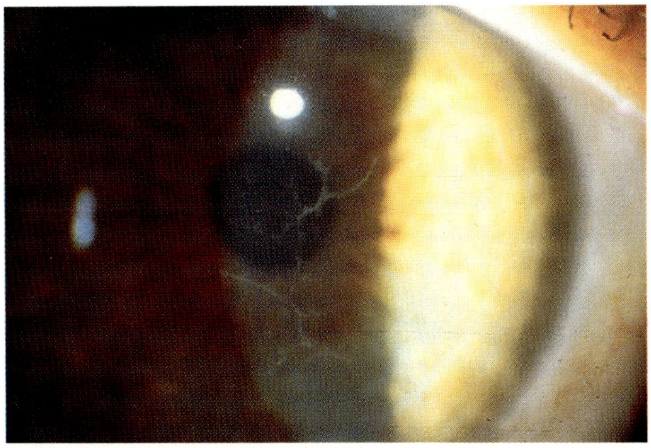

Pseudodendrite.

Figure 3–40. Dendritic epithelial irregularity in soft contact lens wearer.

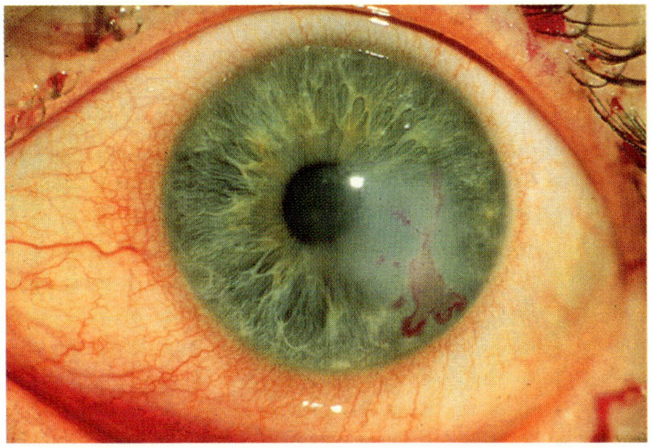

Herpes simplex, stromal keratitis.

Figure 3–41. Well-localized stromal keratitis with recurrent epithelial dendrite due to topical steroid therapy. Classic rose bengal staining pattern of actively infected corneal epithelium at the margin of the ulcer.

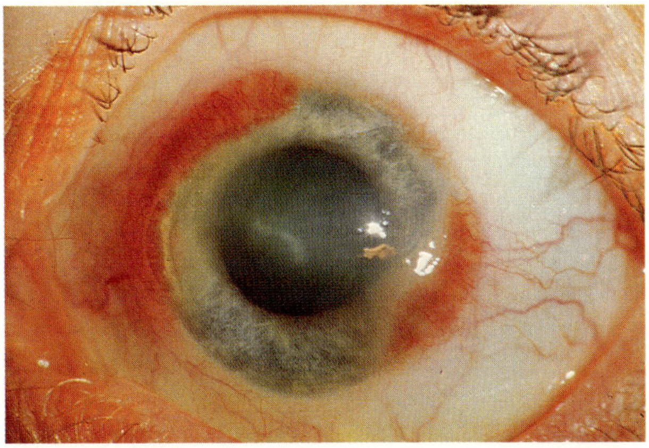

Herpes simplex, stromal keratitis.

Figure 3–42. Diffuse stromal edema and keratitis are seen in association with marked limbal vasculitis. (From Smolin, G., and Thoft, R. (eds.): The Cornea: Scientific Foundations and Clinical Practice. Boston, Little, Brown, and Co., 1983.)

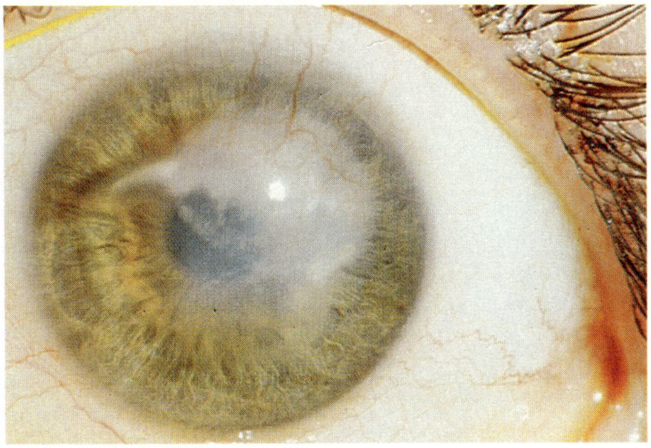

Herpes simplex, stromal keratitis.

Figure 3–43. Necrotic, cheesy infiltrate of stromal keratitis associated with limbal vascularization. (From Langston, D. (ed.): Ocular Viral Disease: International Ophthalmology Clinics, volume 15. Boston, Little, Brown, and Co., 1975.)

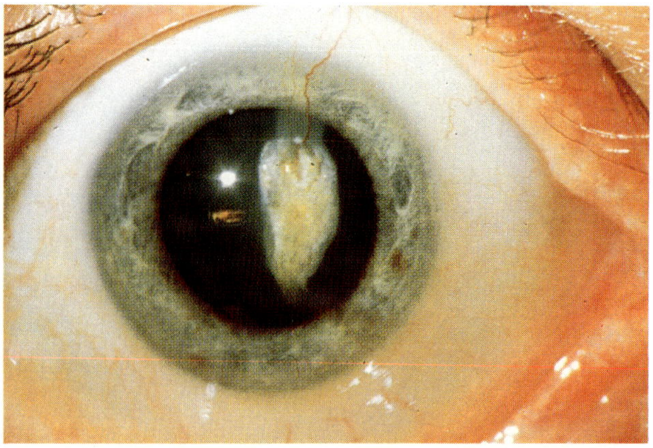

Herpes simplex, stromal keratitis.

Figure 3–44. Dense corneal scarring and deposition of lipid due to chronic stromal keratitis and vascularization.

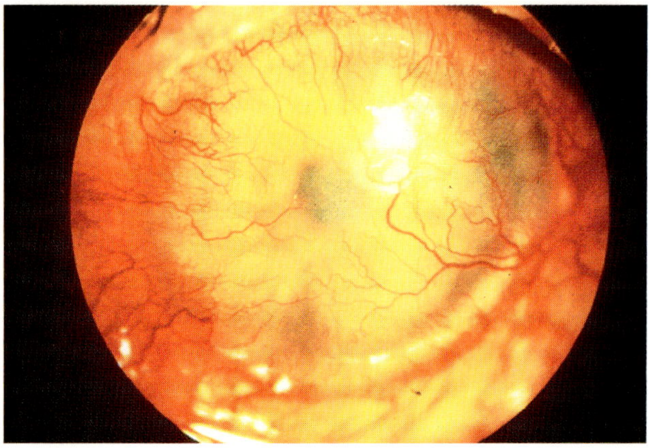

Herpes simplex, stromal keratitis.

Figure 3–45. Irreversible, end stage scarring and vascularization due to recurrent episodes of stromal keratitis.

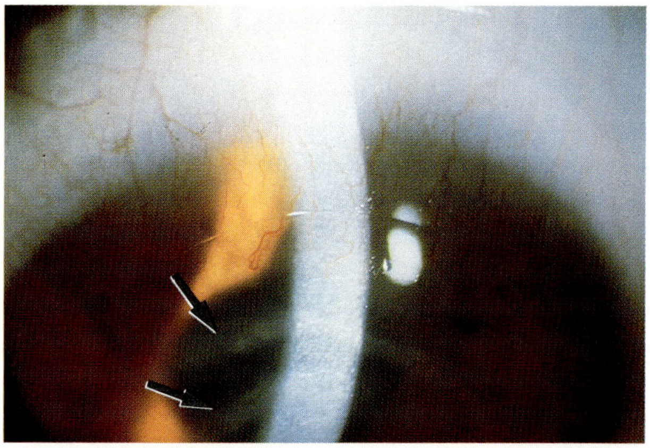

Herpes simplex, stromal keratitis.

Figure 3–46. A double ring infiltrate (arrows) (Wesseley ring) of inflammatory cells in a region of precipitated antigen-antibody complexes is separated from the main stromal lesion by clear cornea. Corneal vascularization is present superiorly.

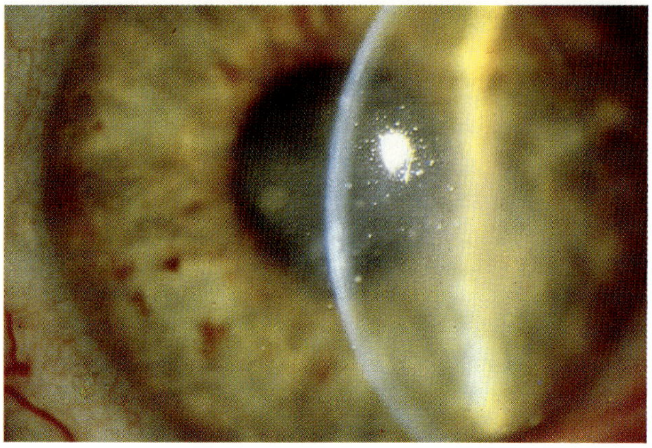

Herpes simplex, disciform keratitis.

Figure 3–47. Large white keratic precipitates in an axial, disciform pattern associated with stromal edema. The remainder of the cornea is clear and compact.

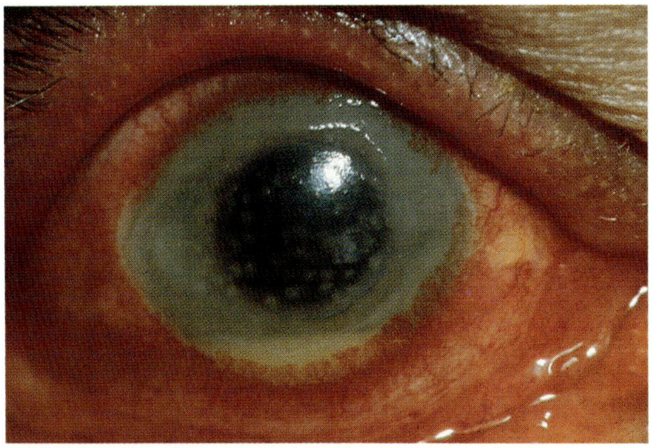

Herpes simplex iridocyclitis.

Figure 3–48. Multiple large white keratic precipitates and stromal edema with an intense anterior chamber reaction and hypopyon.

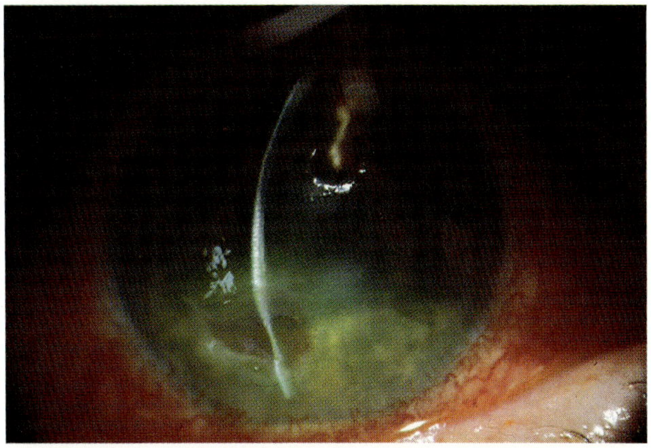

Herpes simplex keratitis, metaherpetic ulcer with perforation.

Figure 3–49. Persistent epithelial defect in anesthetic cornea of patient with recurrent epithelial herpes keratitis with sterile ulceration, perforation, and flat anterior chamber.

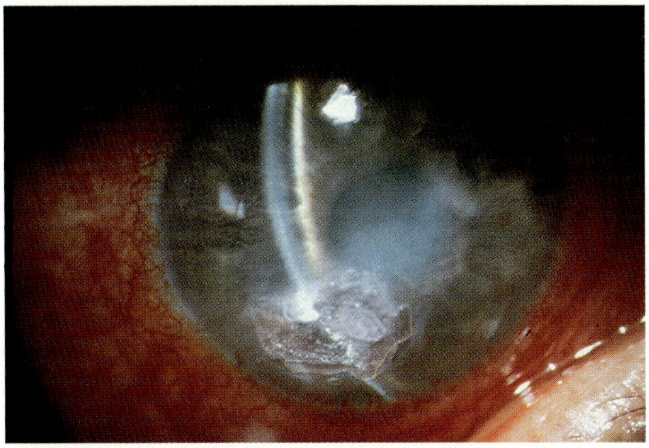

Herpes simplex keratitis, s/p application of cyanoacrylate glue.

Figure 3–50. Same patient as in Figure 3–49 following application of cyanoacrylate glue. The anterior chamber reformed within minutes.

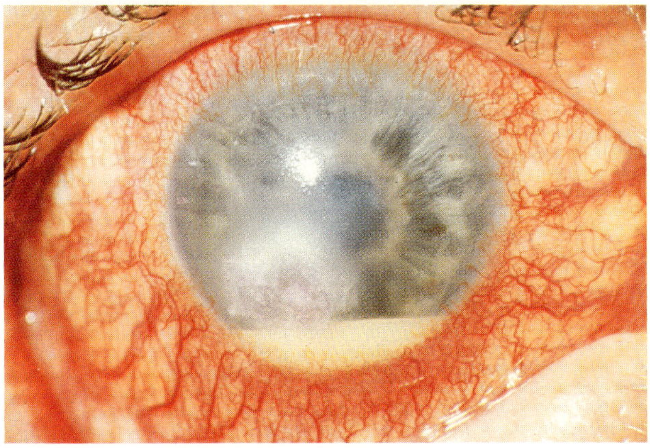

Herpes simplex keratitis, secondary bacterial superinfection.

Figure 3–51. Three months later the cornea became secondarily infected with *Serratia marcescens* with corneal infiltrate adjacent to the glue and secondary hypopyon.

Herpes simplex keratitis, peripheral vascularization.

Figure 3–52. Advanced peripheral vascularization due to presence of cyanoacrylate glue and healed bacterial keratitis.

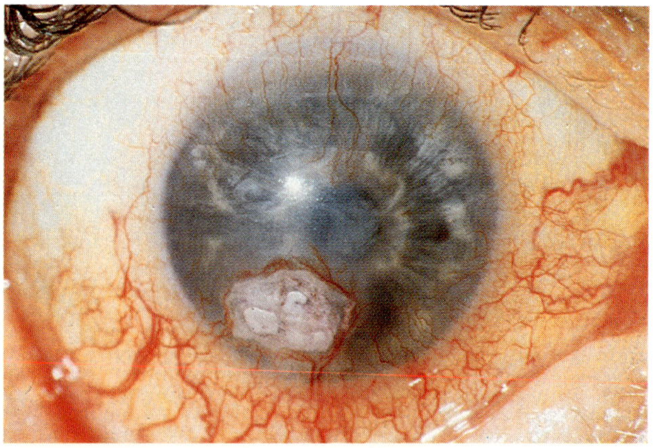

Herpes simplex keratitis, peripheral vascularization.

Figure 3–53. Six months after application of glue, removal of glue reveals the cornea is tectonically stable and well vascularized. A mature lens is present.

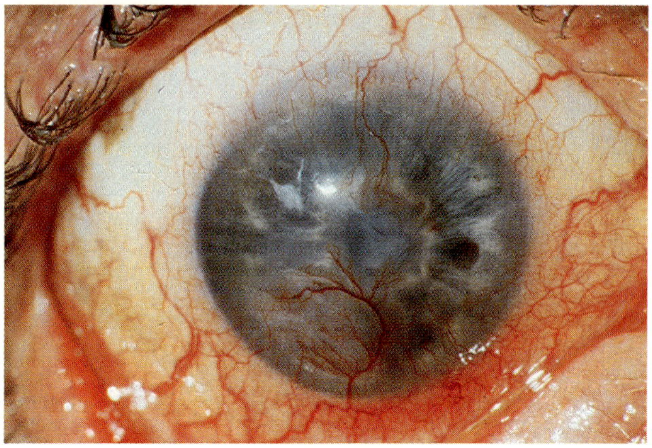

4

Allergy

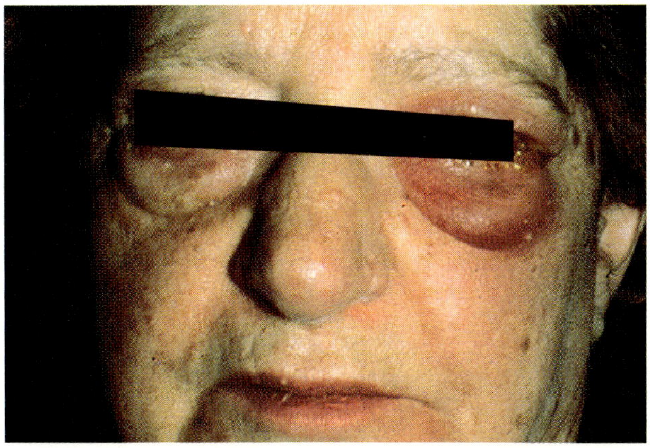

Medication allergy.

Figure 4–1. Marked lid edema and erythema associated with neomycin allergy.

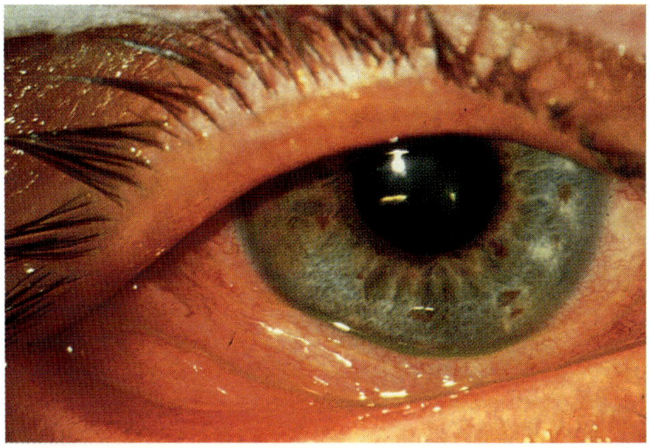

Medication allergy.

Figure 4–2. Typical conjunctival swelling and erythema in same patient shown in Figure 4–1.

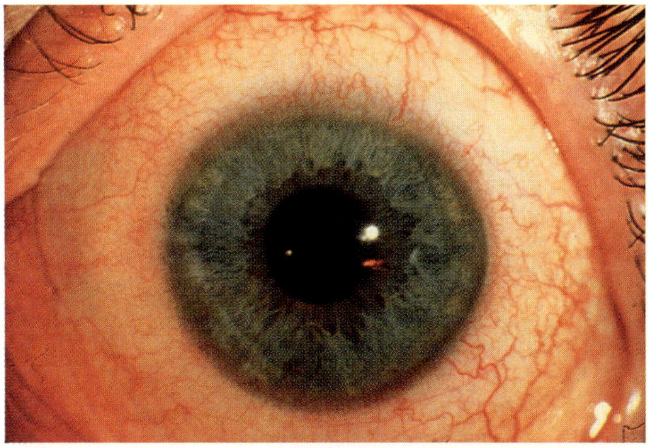

Thimerosal sensitivity.

Figure 4–3. Nonspecific, diffuse conjunctival erythema in soft contact lens wearer using contact lens solutions containing thimerosal.

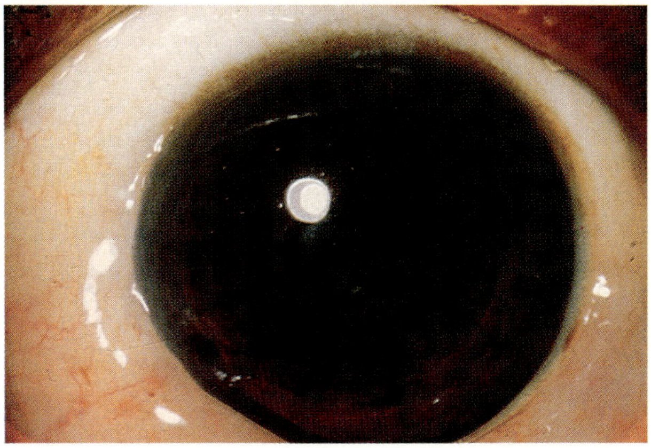

"Hay fever" conjunctivitis.

Figure 4–4. Diffuse conjunctival edema with minimal injection in patient with ragweed allergies.

Atopic keratoconjunctivitis.

Figure 4–5. Thickened, scaling skin and lids with diffuse conjunctival injection associated with atopy.

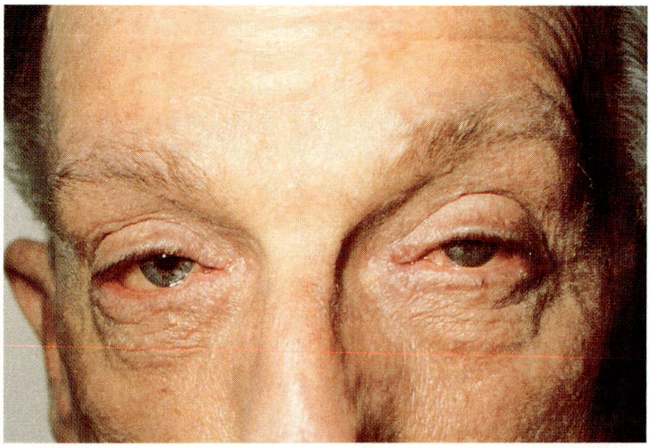

Atopic keratoconjunctivitis.

Figure 4–6. High magnification appearance of characteristic lid induration and lichenification of chronic atopic dermatitis.

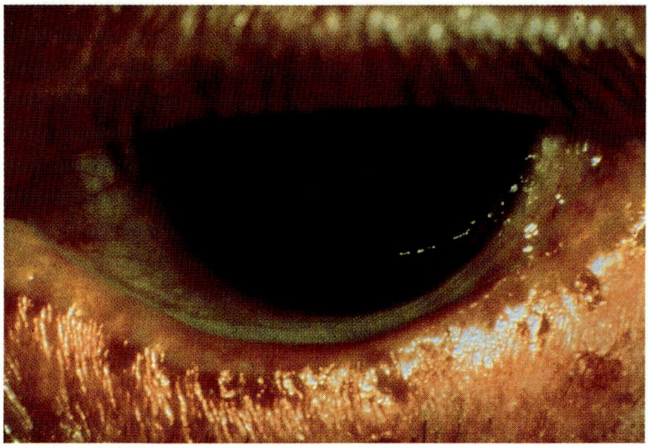

Atopic keratoconjunctivitis.

Figure 4–7. Chronic palpebral and bulbar conjunctival injection with early symblepharon formation (arrow) medially.

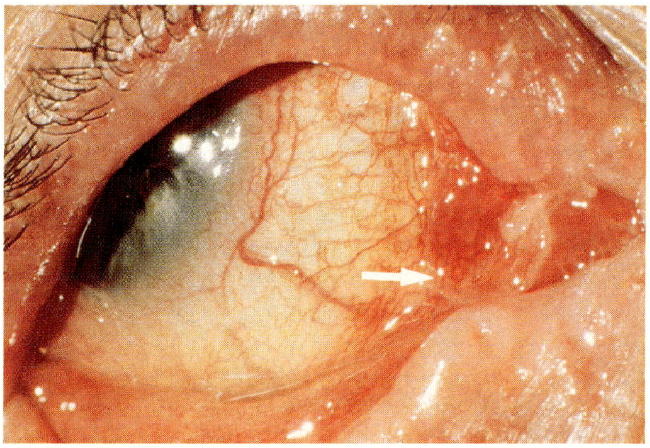

Atopic keratoconjunctivitis.

Figure 4–8. Persistent epithelial defect associated with atopy that was unresponsive to topical lubrication and retinoid therapy.

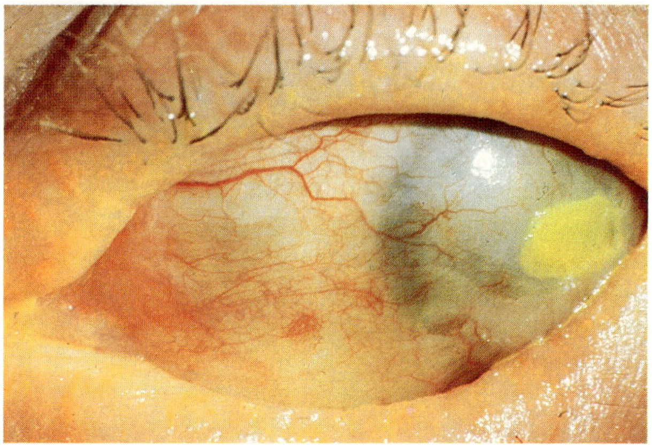

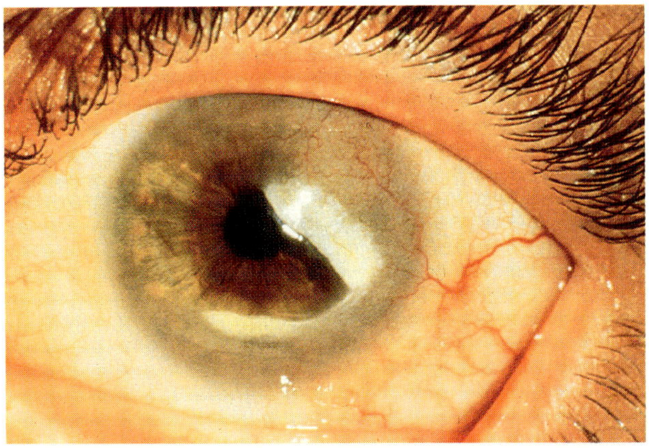

Atopic keratoconjunctivitis.

Figure 4–9. Corneal vascularization and secondary lipid keratopathy associated with atopy.

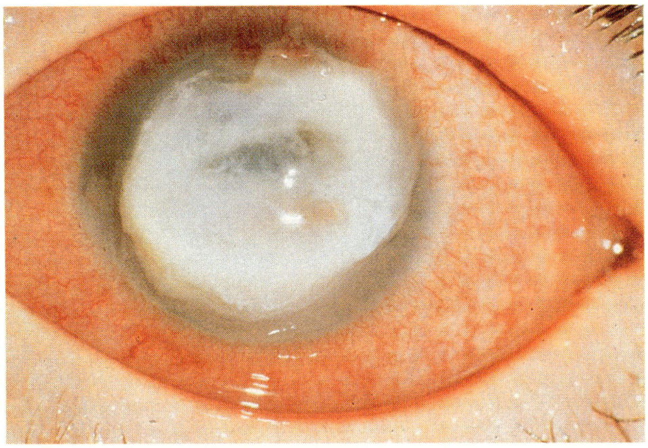

Atopic keratoconjunctivitis.

Figure 4–10. Persistent epithelial defect due to atopy has resulted in sterile stromal ulceration with impending perforation.

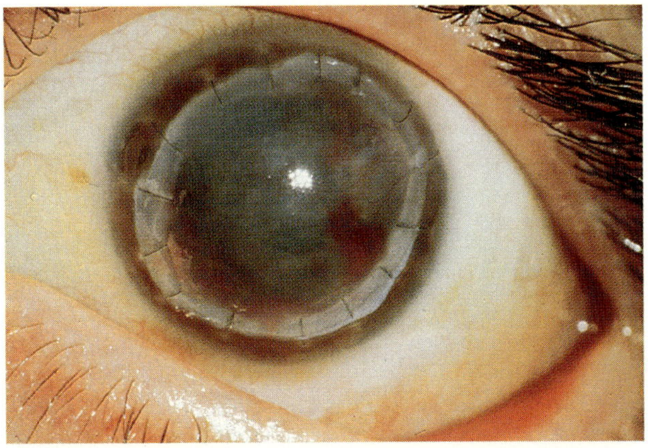

Atopic keratoconjunctivitis.

Figure 4–11. Same patient shown in Figure 4–10 following tectonic lamellar keratoplasty and systemic, psychiatric, and environmental control therapy.

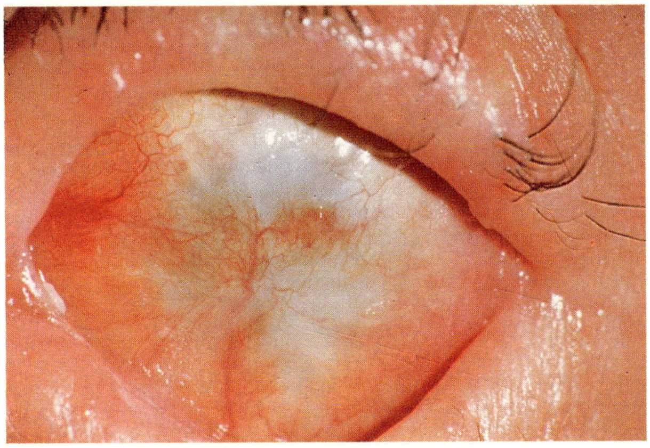

Atopic keratoconjunctivitis.

Figure 4–12. End stage ocular surface scarring following two unsuccessful penetrating keratoplasties for persistent epithelial defects due to atopy.

Atopic keratoconjunctivitis.

Figure 4–13. Severe keratoconjunctivitis with pannus formation.

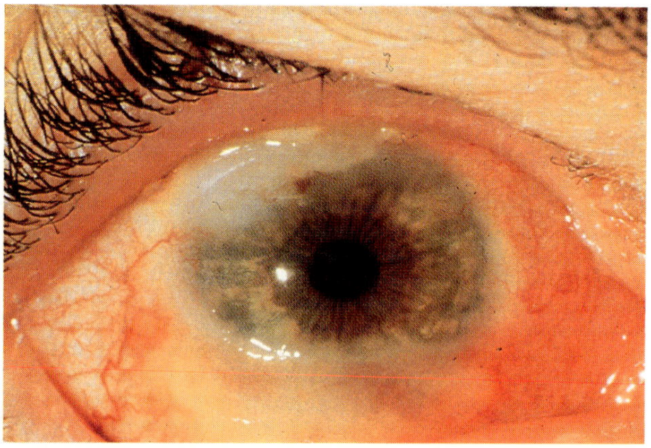

Atopic keratoconjunctivitis.

Figure 4–14. Same patient shown in Figure 4–12 with virtually complete resolution of corneal pannus following appropriate multidisciplinary therapy.

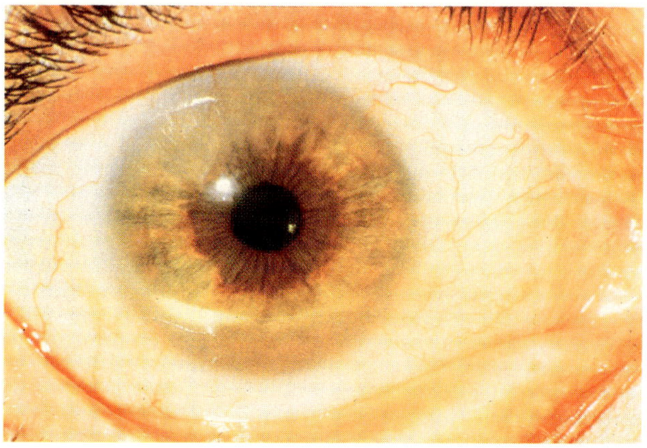

Vernal keratoconjunctivitis, palpebral form.

Figure 4–15. Giant papillary excrescences or "cobblestones" on the upper tarsal conjunctiva associated with abundant fibrin accumulation.

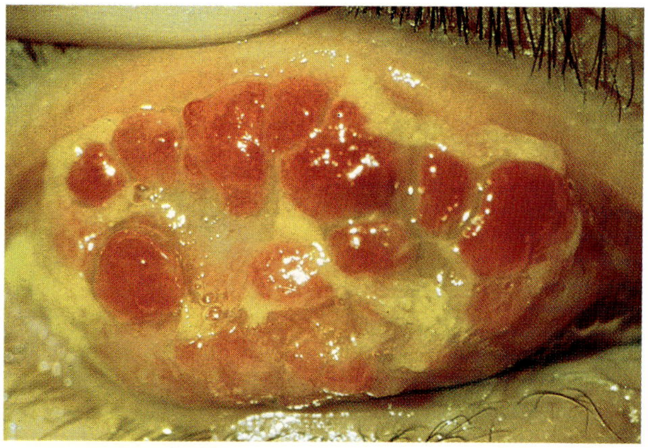

Vernal keratoconjunctivitis, palpebral form.

Figure 4–16. Corneal scar formation in region of previous "shield ulcers." The superior lesion is characteristically positioned and shaped, whereas the inferior lesion is somewhat atypically located.

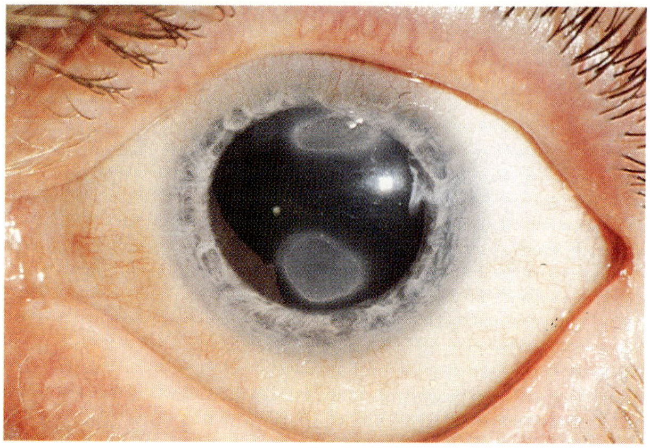

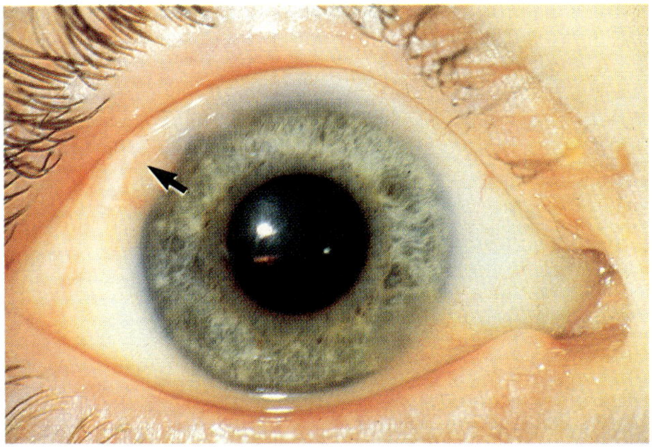

Vernal keratoconjunctivitis, limbal form.

Figure 4–17. Pink, elevated gelatinous limbal papillary lesions (arrow) are present at 10:00. Note the limbal vascularization between 4:00 and 5:00.

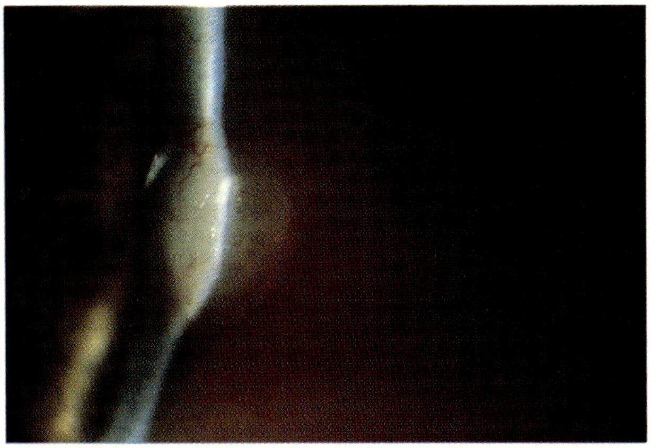

Vernal keratoconjunctivitis, limbal form.

Figure 4–18. High magnification, slit lamp appearance of large elevated limbal papilla.

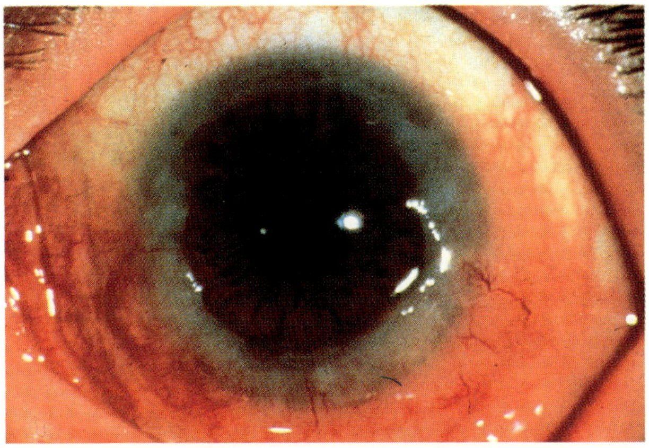

Vernal keratoconjunctivitis, limbal form.

Figure 4–19. Advanced case with 360° extension of limbal papillary reaction.

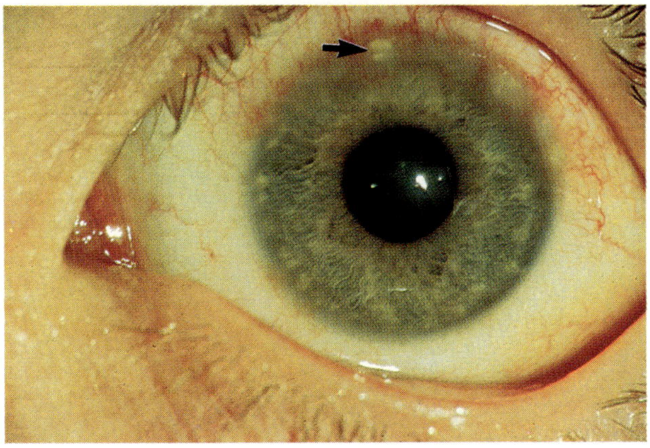

Vernal keratoconjunctivitis, limbal form.

Figure 4–20. Raised masses with whitish chalklike excrescences or Trantas dots (arrow) can be seen within the limbal papilla.

5

Systemic Associations

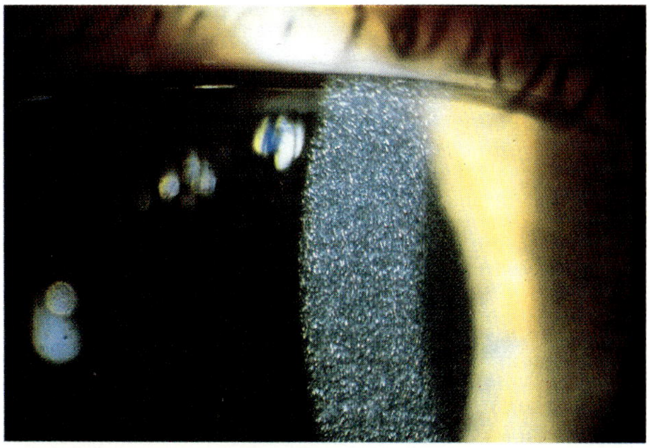

Cystinosis.

Figure 5–1. Dense, uniformly distributed accumulation of glistening, polychromatic, needlelike to rectangular crystals in the anterior stroma of patient with adult cystinosis.

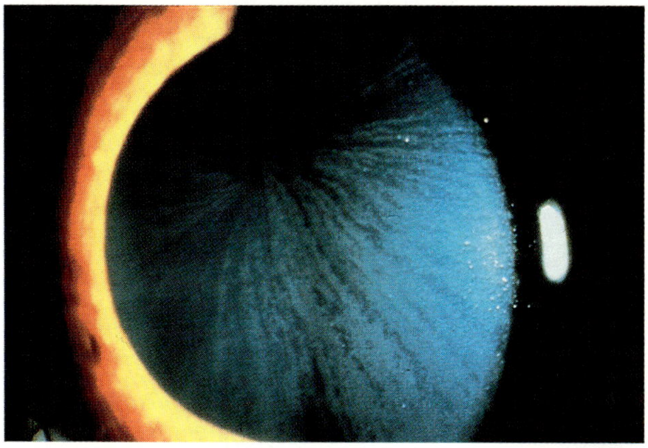

Fabry's disease.

Figure 5–2. Fine, whirllike superficial corneal opacification in female carrier of Fabry's disease. The corneal appearance is indistinguishable from the corneal opacities found after administration of chloroquine or amiodarone.

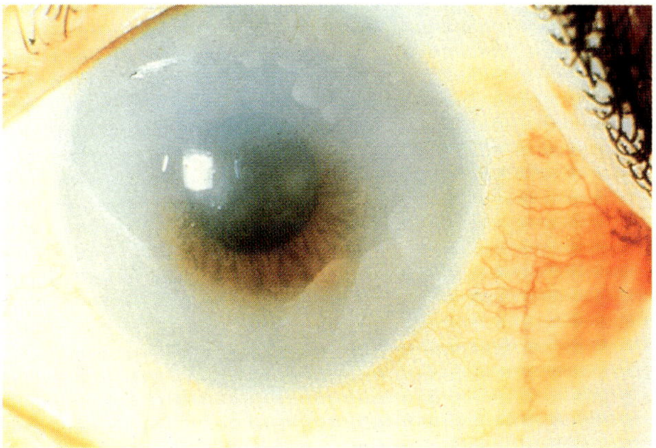

Mucopolysaccharidosis.

Figure 5–3. Corneal haze and edematous thickening are much more marked in the peripheral cornea in this patient with Hurler's syndrome.

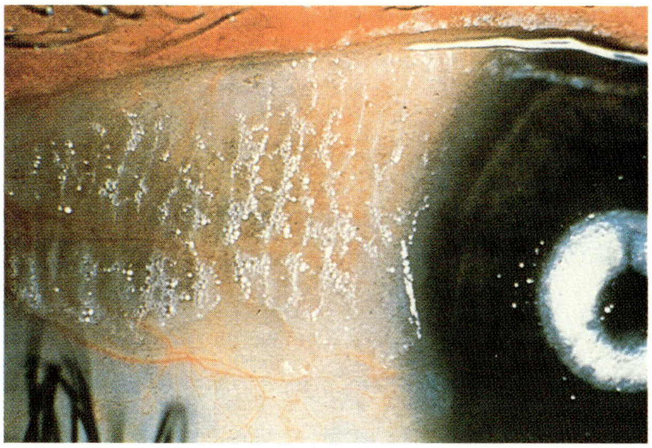

Hypovitaminosis A, Bitot's spot.

Figure 5–4. Extensive temporal bulbar Bitot's spot consisting of a large, light gray plaque with rough, foamy texture.

Hypovitaminosis A, corneal ulceration.

Figure 5–5. Persistent epithelial defect associated with corneal xerosis has resulted in circumscribed area of corneal necrosis and thinning inferiorly. (From Arch. Ophthalmol. 100:953, 1982. Copyright 1982, American Medical Association.)

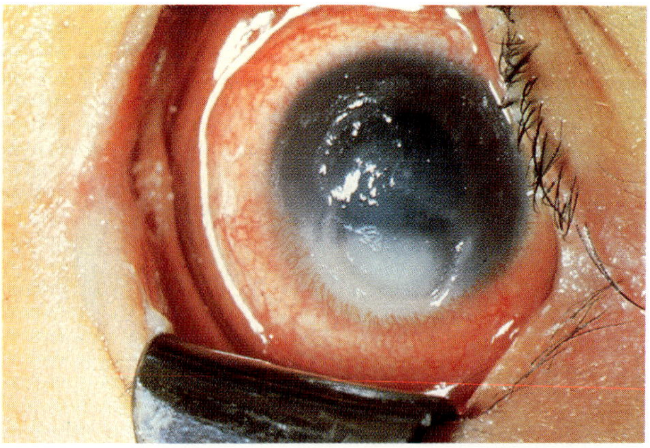

Hypovitaminosis A, corneal ulceration.

Figure 5–6. Same patient shown in Figure 5–5 two days later and two hours before death. The lower two thirds of the cornea is opaque and necrotic in appearance. Gram-negative rods were present on histopathologic examination. (From Arch. Ophthalmol. 100:953, 1982. Copyright 1982, American Medical Association.)

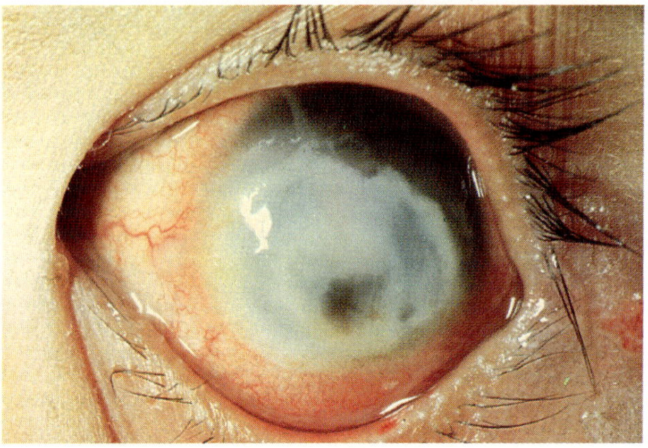

Neurotrophic ulcer secondary to trigeminal palsy.

Figure 5–7. Classic indolent ulcer of corneal denervation with inferior location, horizontally oval configuration, "heaped up" gray edges of epithelium, and extensive ocular inflammation. (From Smolin, G., and Thoft, R. (eds.): The Cornea: Scientific Foundations and Clinical Practice. Boston, Little, Brown, and Co., 1983, p. 321.)

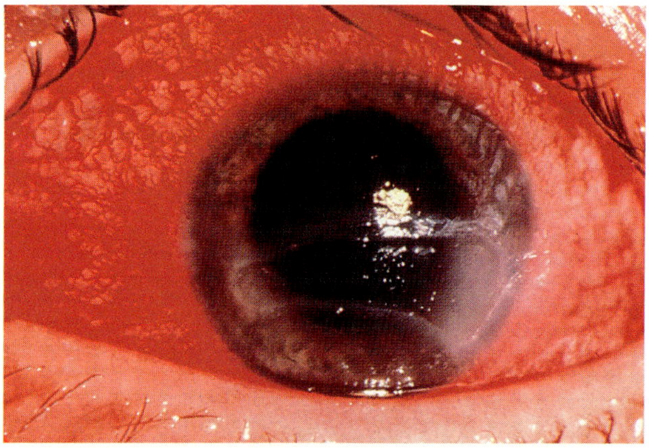

Neurotrophic ulcer secondary to familial dysautonomia.

Figure 5–8. Persistent epithelial defect in young girl with Riley-Day syndrome has resulted in secondary sterile corneal ulceration and opacification.

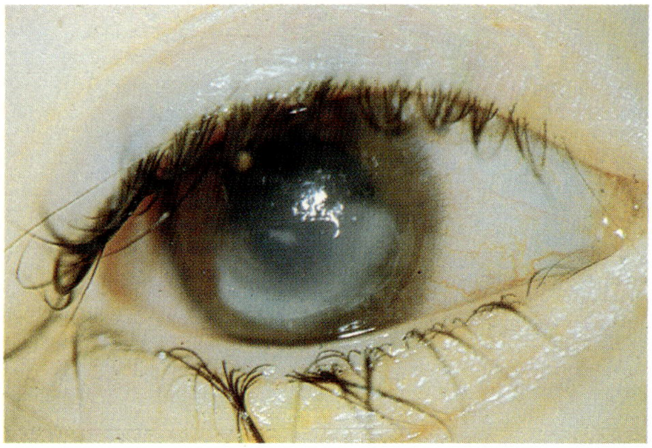

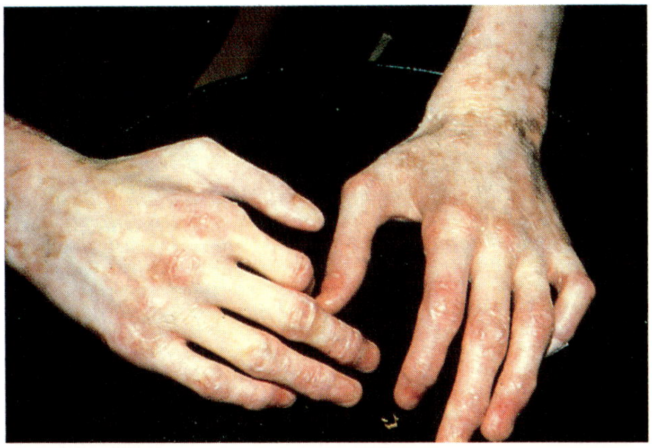

Graft vs. host disease.

Figure 5–9. Typical erythematous cutaneous eruptions with scaling and dermal fibrosis in advanced case of graft vs. host disease.

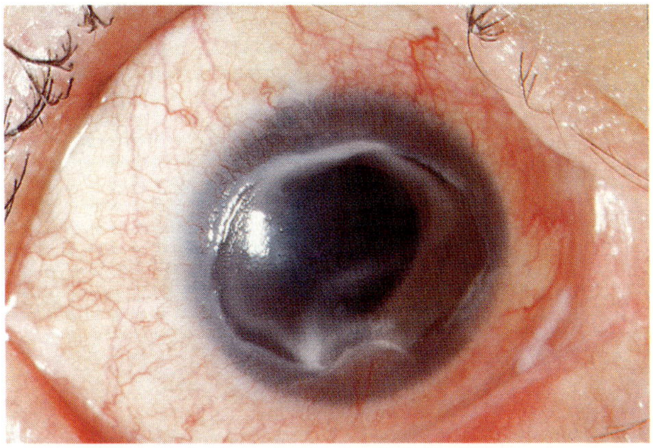

Graft vs. host disease.

Figure 5–10. Persistent epithelial defect with peripheral vascularization in patient shown in Figure 5–9.

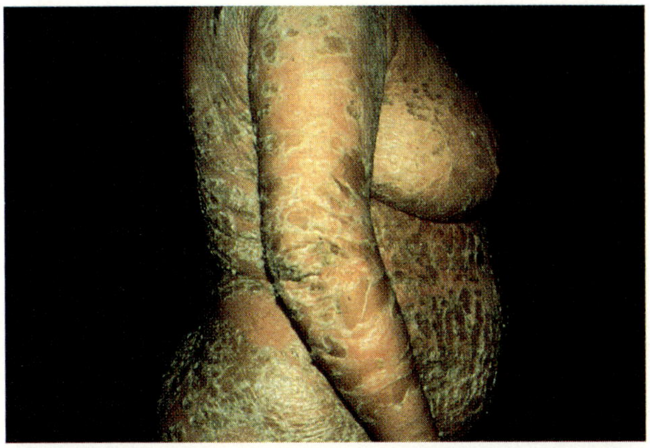

Ichthyosis.

Figure 5–11. Classic dermal appearance of ichthyosis with dry skin and rhomboidal scales with flaky edges.

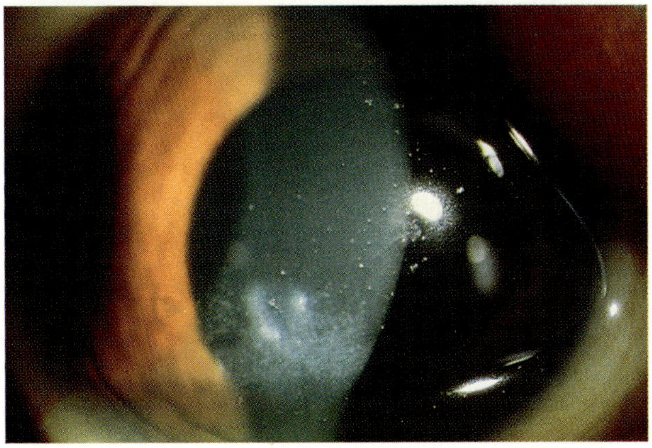

Ichthyosis.

Figure 5–12. Subepithelial infiltrates in the cornea of patient shown in Figure 5–11.

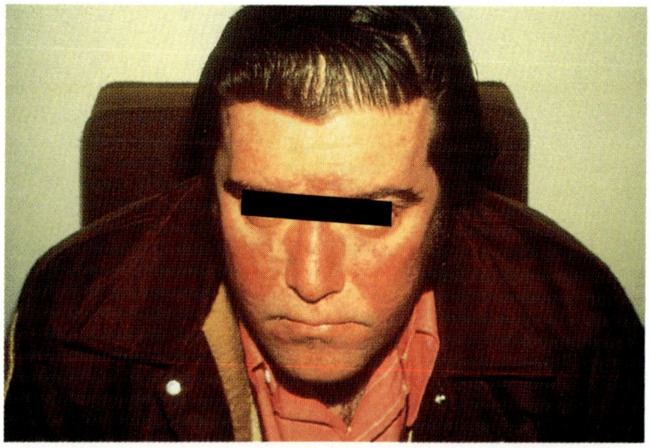

Acne rosacea.

Figure 5–13. Typical distribution of the telangiectatic, erythematous cutaneous eruption of acne rosacea with early thickening of the nasal skin (rhinophyma).

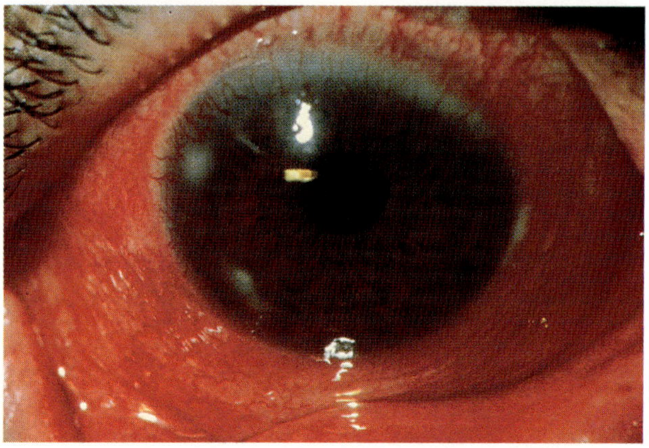

Acne rosacea.

Figure 5–14. Marked meibomitis, peripheral corneal infiltrates, and peripheral vascularization in patient with uncontrolled cutaneous acne rosacea.

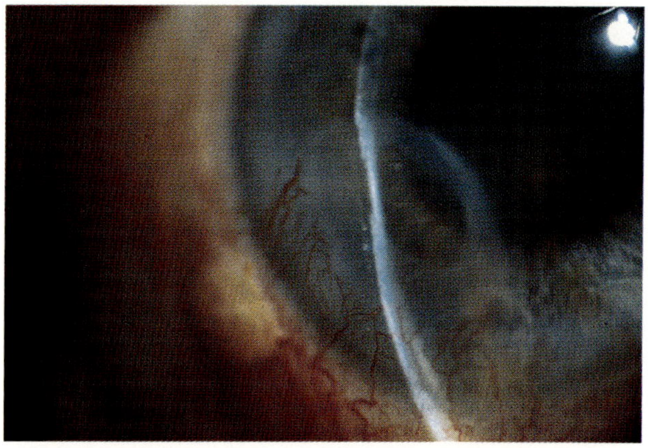

Acne rosacea.

Figure 5–15. Peripheral vascularization, persistent epithelial defect, and corneal thinning in untreated acne rosacea.

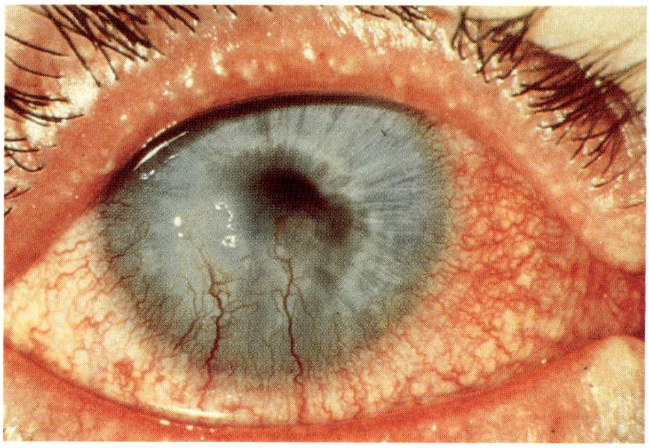

Acne rosacea.

Figure 5–16. Severe inferior pannus formation in patient with chronic acne rosacea and significant blepharitis.

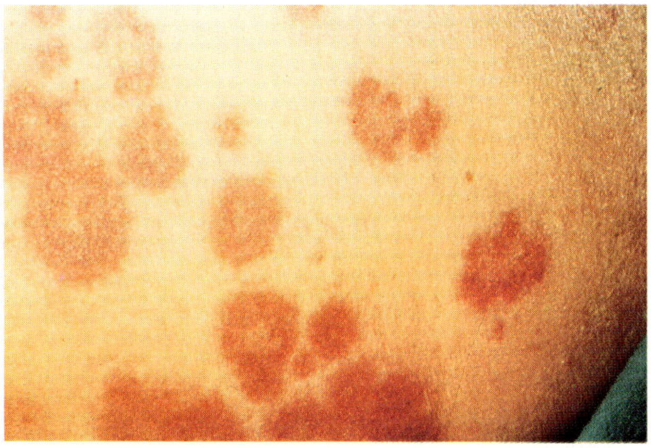

Erythema multiforme (Stevens-Johnson syndrome).

Figure 5–17. Typical skin eruptions with raised, erythematous lesions with characteristic "bull's eye" appearance due to variable pigmentation.

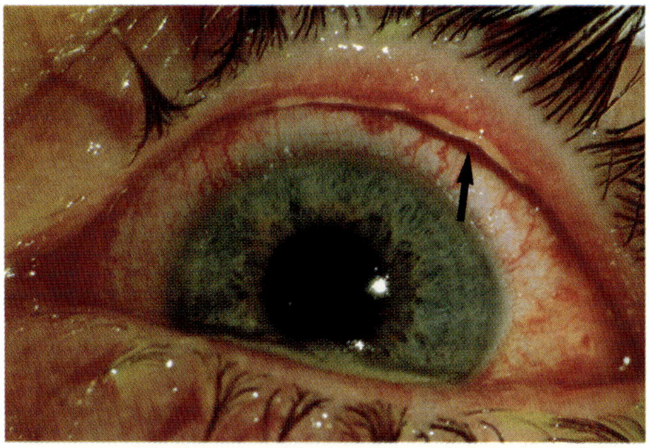

Erythema multiforme.

Figure 5–18. Classic mucopurulent blepharoconjunctivitis associated with active skin eruptions. Note the prominent meibomitis and the edge of a large pseudomembrane beneath the upper lid (arrow).

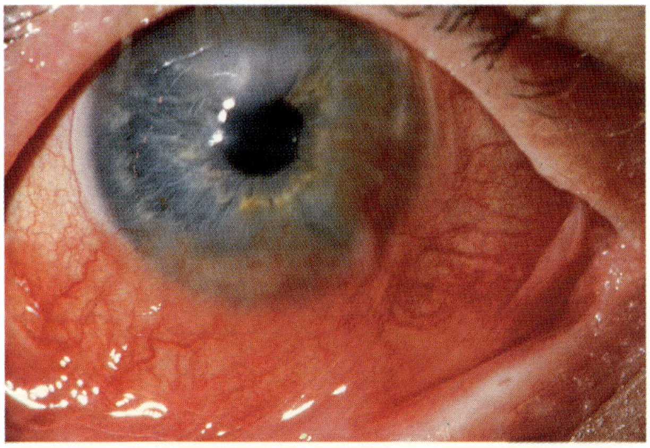

Erythema multiforme.

Figure 5–19. Advanced conjunctival scarring has produced extensive symblepharon inferiorly with obliteration of the inferior fornix, inferior corneal pannus, and superior corneal pannus with early corneal opacification. This appearance is indistinguishable from cicatricial pemphigoid, Foster stage III (Figures 5–25, 5–33, 5–35.)

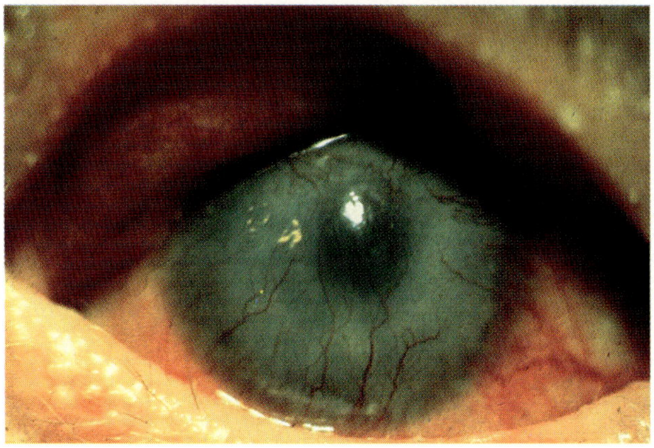

Erythema multiforme.

Figure 5–20. End stage, extensive conjunctival scarring and pannus following resolution of cutaneous disease. Note the cicatricial scarring of the superior tarsal conjunctiva.

Cicatricial pemphigoid.

Figure 5–21. Typical oral mucosal lesions, with epithelial erosion and subepithelial fibrosis in patient with oral mucosal and ocular cicatricial pemphigoid.

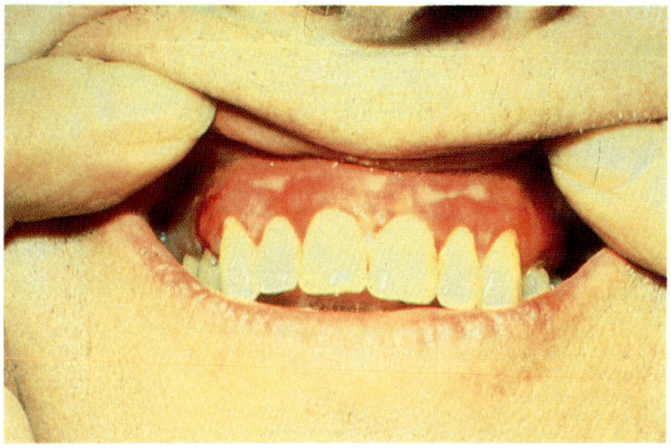

Cicatricial pemphigoid, Foster stage I.

Figure 5–22. Fine white subepithelial fibrotic striae and "feltwork" pattern of conjunctival scarring associated with chronic conjunctival injection and mucoid discharge.

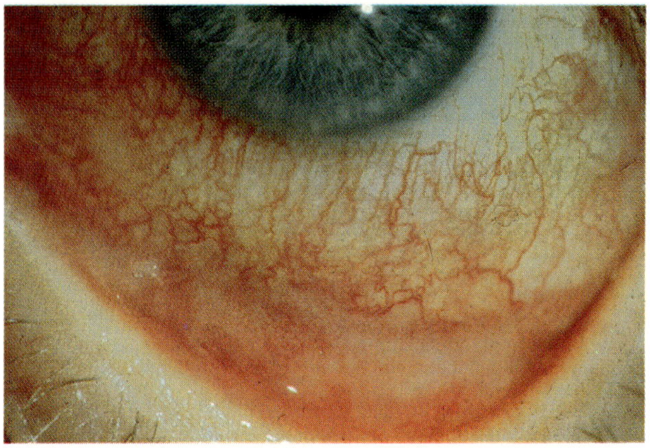

Cicatricial pemphigoid, Foster stage I.

Figure 5–23. Subepithelial fibrosis with scarring in upper tarsal conjunctiva.

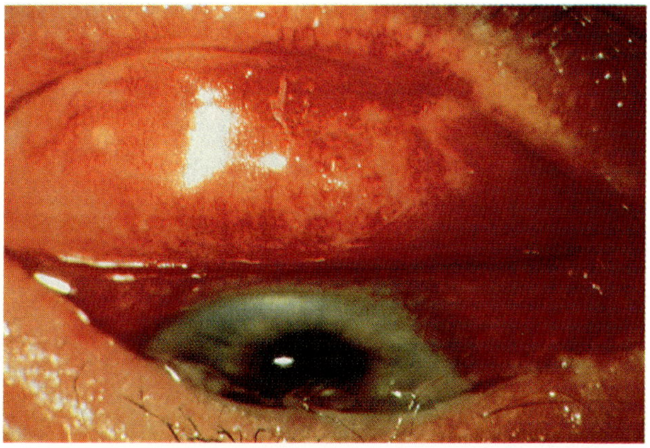

Cicatricial pemphigoid, Foster stage II.

Figure 5–24. Subepithelial fibrosis is associated with foreshortening of the inferior conjunctival cul-de-sac.

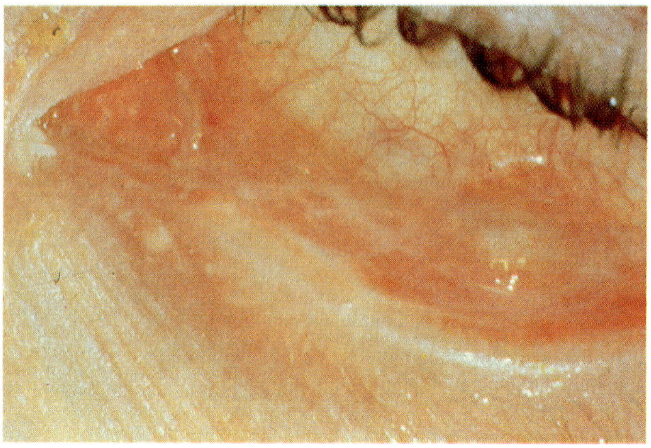

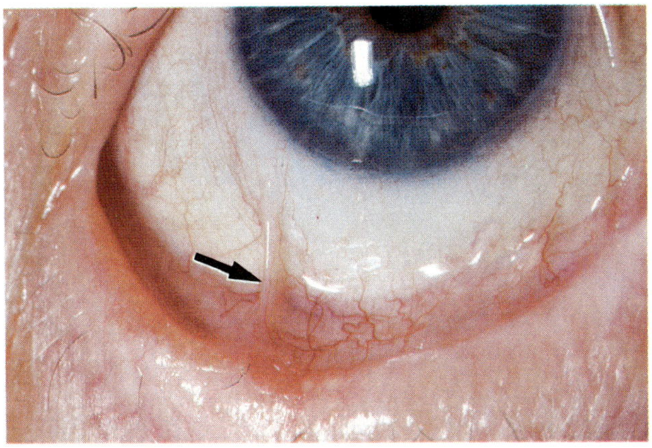

Cicatricial pemphigoid, Foster stage III.

Figure 5–25. Continued formation and contraction of subconjunctival connective tissue has resulted in symblepharon (arrow) formation. Note the extensive subepithelial fibrosis and foreshortened, blunted inferior fornix.

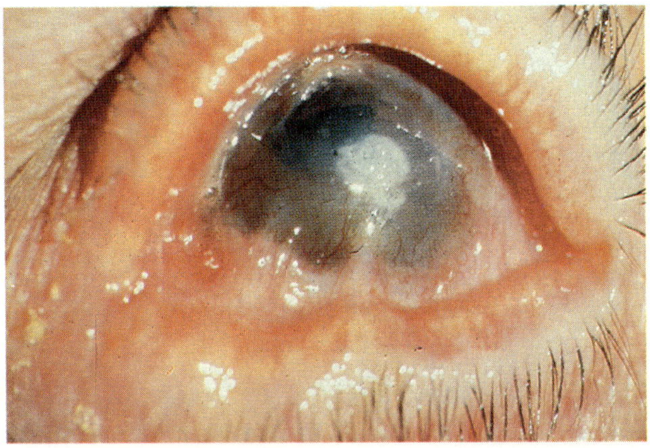

Cicatricial pemphigoid, Foster stage IV.

Figure 5–26. End stage disease with ankyloblepharon (adhesion of lids to globe), extensive symblepharon, severe sicca, and advanced corneal vascularization.

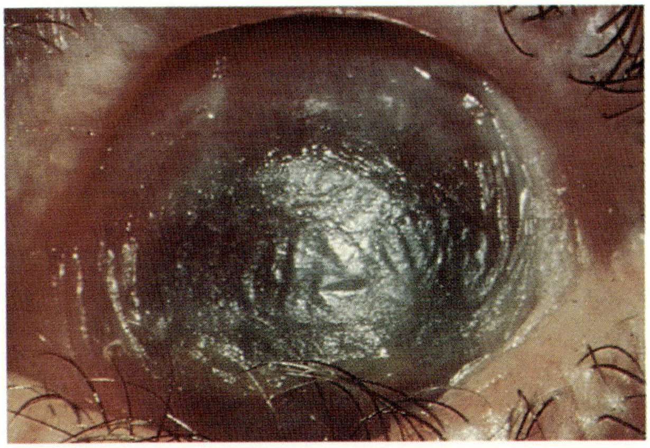

Cicatricial pemphigoid, Foster stage IV.

Figure 5–27. End stage disease with total corneal keratinization and opacification.

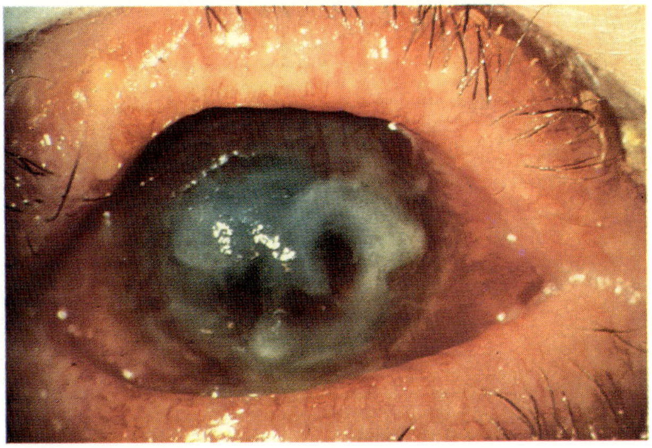

Cicatricial pemphigoid, secondary bacterial superinfection.

Figure 5–28. Foster stage III cicatricial pemphigoid with persistent epithelial defect and secondary bacterial superinfection with corneal necrosis and descemetocele formation.

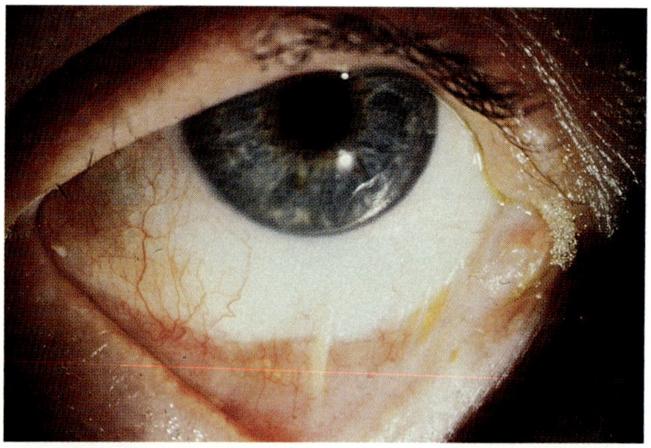

Cicatricial pemphigoid, Mondino stage I.

Figure 5–29. Less than 25 per cent conjunctival shrinkage of conjunctival fornix and symblepharon of the inferior fornix. (Courtesy of Dr. Bartly Mondino.)

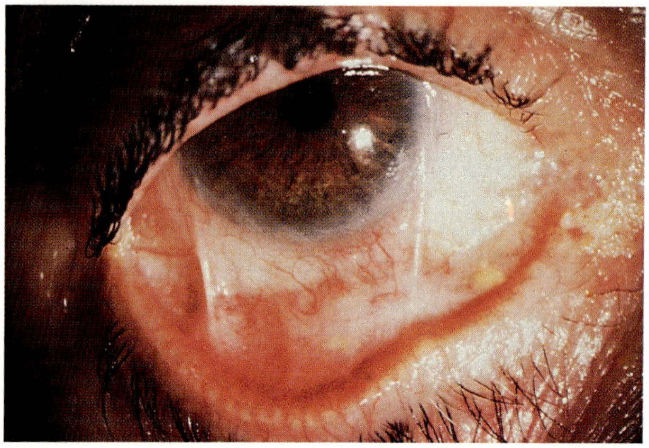

Cicatricial pemphigoid, Mondino stage II.

Figure 5–30. Conjunctival shrinkage is between 25 and 50 percent, with prominent symblephara. (Courtesy of Dr. Bartly Mondino.)

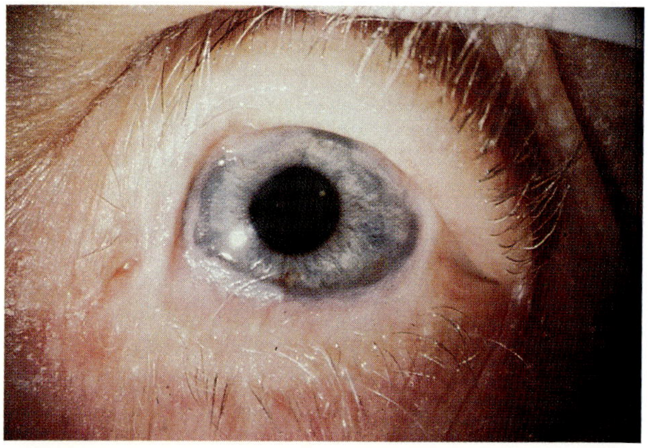

Cicatricial pemphigoid, Mondino stage III.

Figure 5–31. Severe shrinkage of the inferior fornix (approximately 75 per cent) with severe symblephara. The upper fornix is still present. (Courtesy of Dr. Bartly Mondino.)

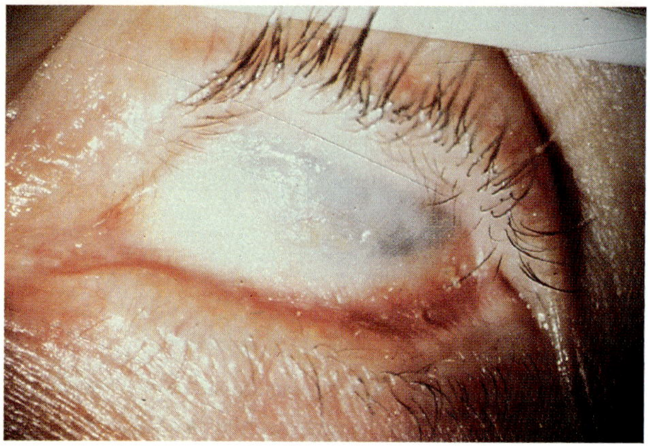

Cicatricial pemphigoid, Mondino stage IV.

Figure 5–32. End stage disease with obliteration of the conjunctival fornices and keratinized ocular surface. (Courtesy of Dr. Bartly Mondino.)

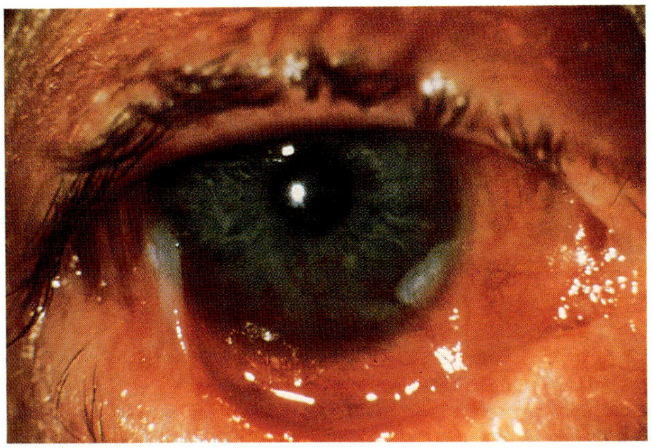

Cicatricial pemphigoid.

Figure 5–33. Foster stage III disease with marked conjunctival inflammation prior to immunosuppressive therapy.

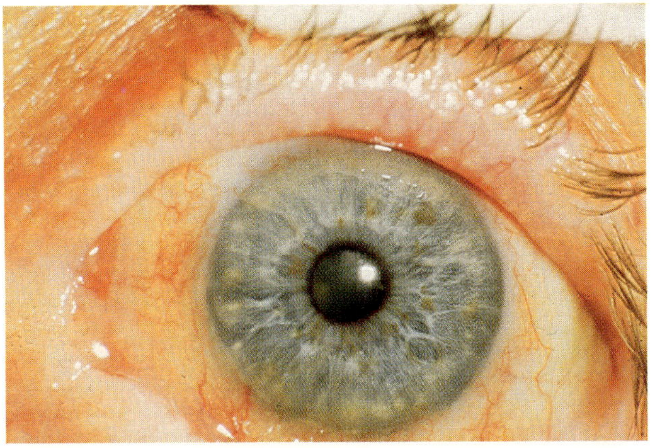

Cicatricial pemphigoid.

Figure 5–34. Same patient shown in Figure 5–33 after two months of therapy with systemic cyclophosphamide showing marked reduction in conjunctival activity.

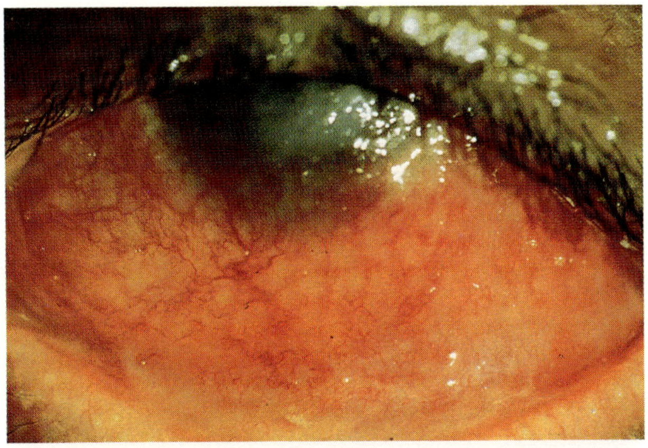

Cicatricial pemphigoid.

Figure 5–35. Foster stage III disease with marked conjunctival activity and inferior keratopathy prior to immunosuppressive therapy.

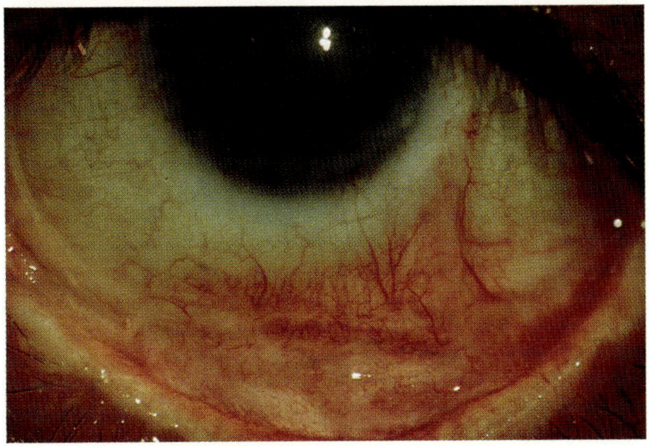

Cicatricial pemphigoid.

Figure 5–36. Same patient shown in Figure 5–35 after two and a half months of systemic immunosuppressive therapy. Note marked resolution of both conjunctival and corneal activity.

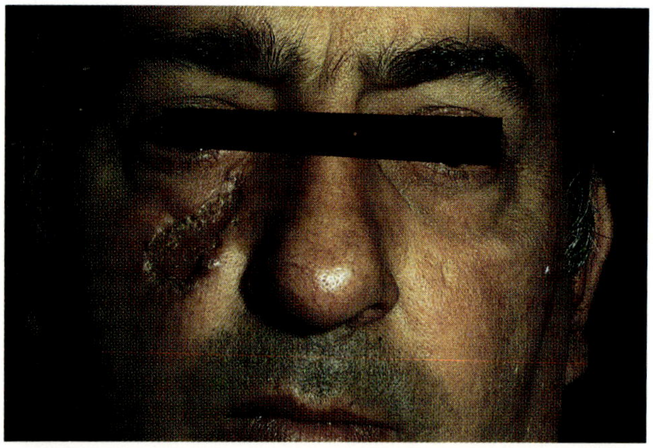

Wegener's granulomatosis.

Figure 5–37. Diagnosis in this case was established by biopsy of cutaneous lesion on right cheek.

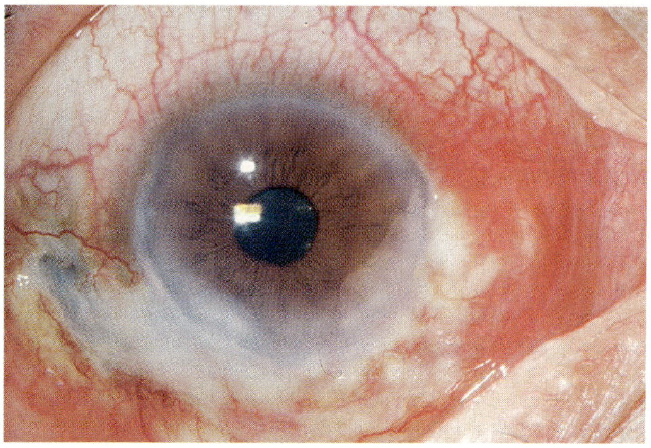

Wegener's granulomatosis.

Figure 5–38. Peripheral ulcerative keratitis with marked associated scleritis in patient shown in Figure 5–37.

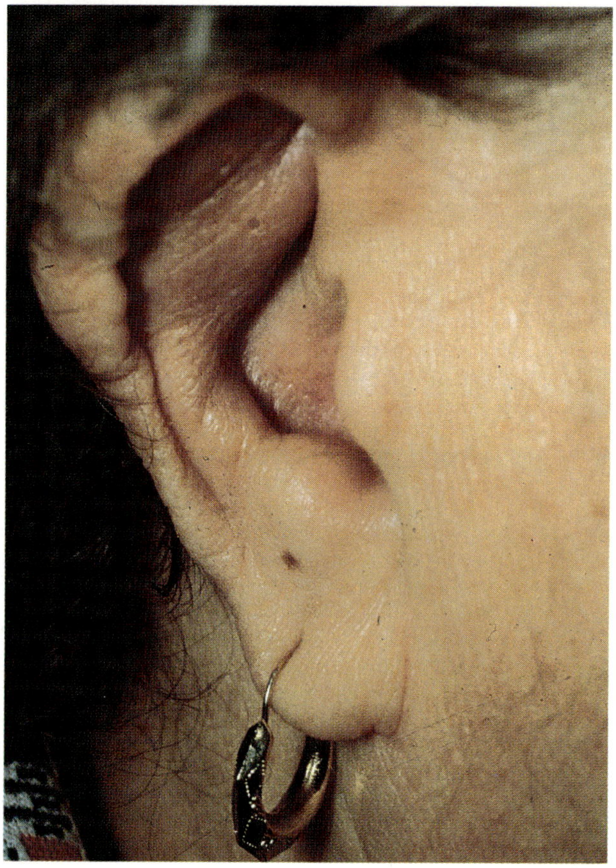

Relapsing polychondritis.

Figure 5–39. Soft and atrophic external ear due to cartilage destruction in patient with chronic relapsing polychondritis.

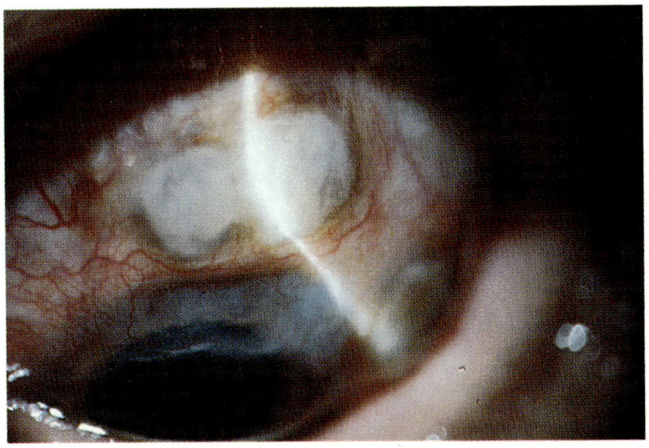

Relapsing polychondritis.

Figure 5–40. Extensive scleritis and peripheral ulcerative keratitis in patient shown in Figure 5–39.

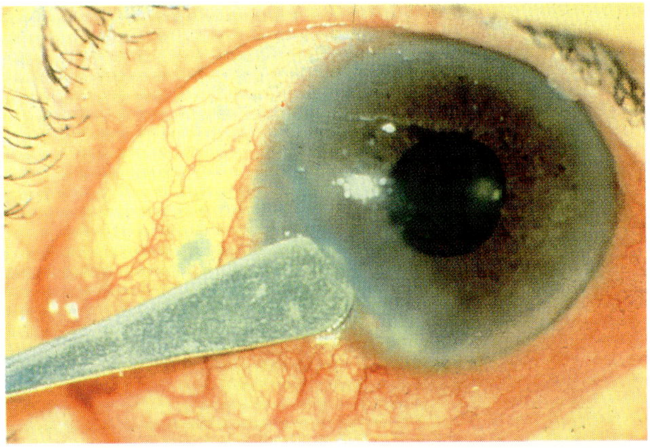

Mooren's ulceration.

Figure 5–41. Peripheral ulcerative keratitis with scleral sparing (in contrast to Figures 5–38 and 5–40) and typical undermined advancing border in patient with bilateral disease.

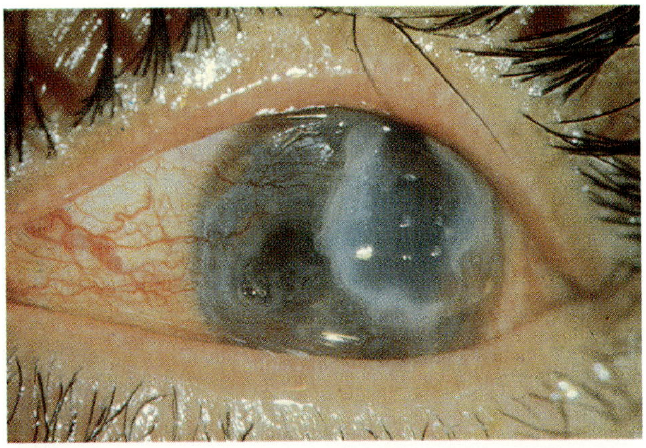

Mooren's ulceration.

Figure 5–42. Advanced 360° involvement of peripheral ulcerative keratitis with axial extension, especially temporally. Prominent vasculature and descemetocele are present temporally.

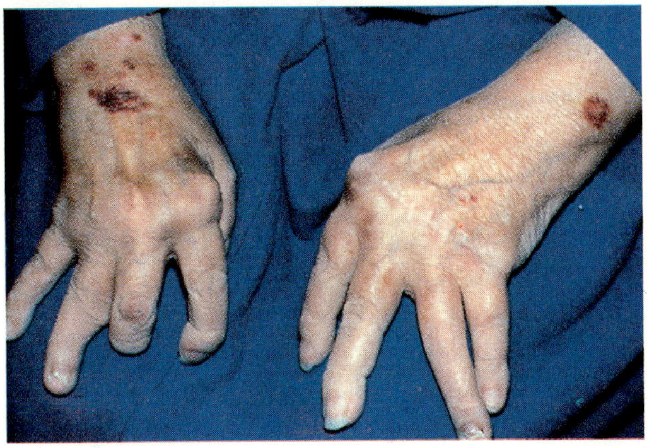

Rheumatoid arthritis.

Figure 5–43. Typical hand deformity of patient with advanced rheumatoid arthritis.

Rheumatoid arthritis, keratoconjunctivitis sicca.

Figure 5–44. Classic rose bengal staining pattern of eye with severe keratoconjunctivitis sicca. Rose bengal staining is prominent in the inferior cornea and conjunctiva in the interpalpebral fissure.

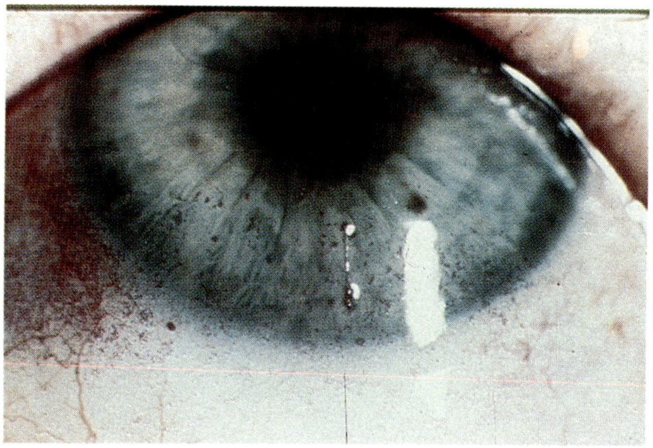

Rheumatoid arthritis, filamentary keratitis.

Figure 5–45. Advanced filamentary keratitis associated with severe keratoconjunctivitis sicca.

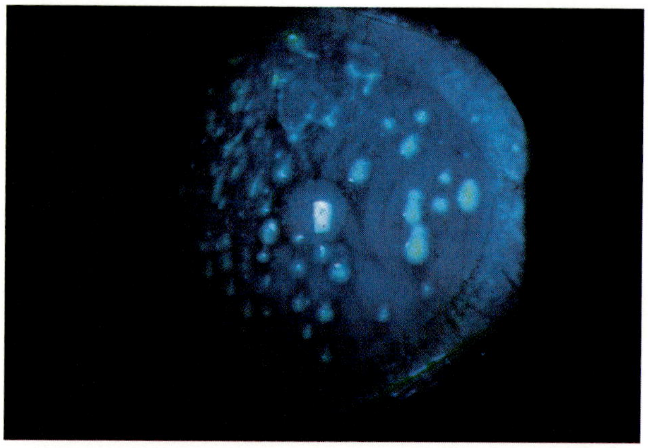

Rheumatoid arthritis, sterile corneal ulceration.

Figure 5–46. Small, persistent central epithelial defect has resulted in sterile ulceration and perforation in a relatively quiet eye.

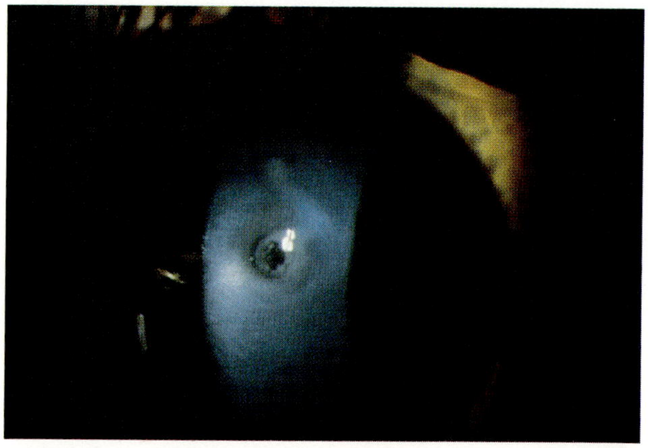

Rheumatoid arthritis, sterile corneal ulceration.

Figure 5–47. A large, persistent epithelial defect has resulted in a large area of sterile ulceration, perforation, iris prolapse, and flat anterior chamber.

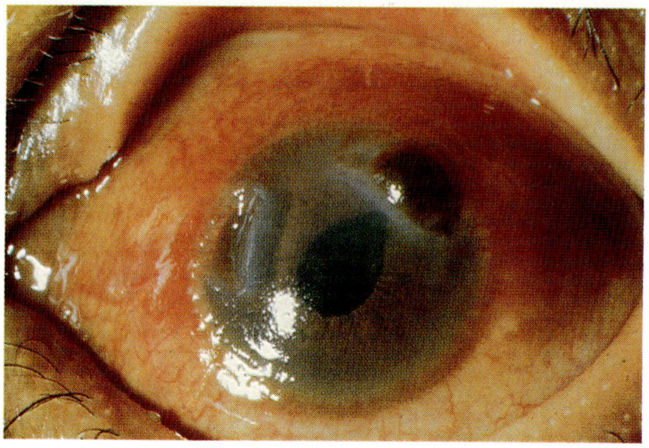

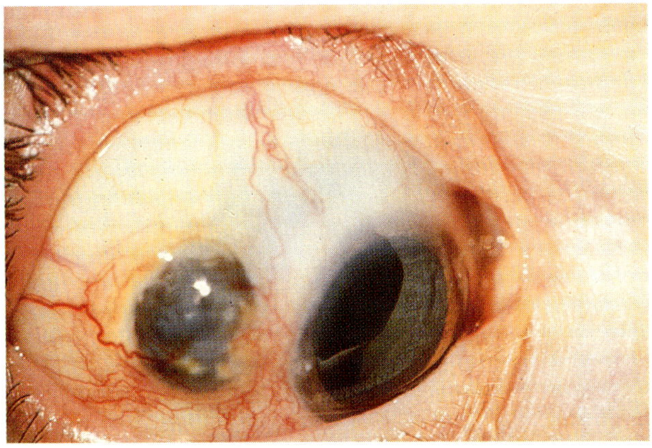

Rheumatoid arthritis, scleromalacia perforans.

Figure 5–48. Uveal prolapse is present temporally following dissolution of overlying sclera.

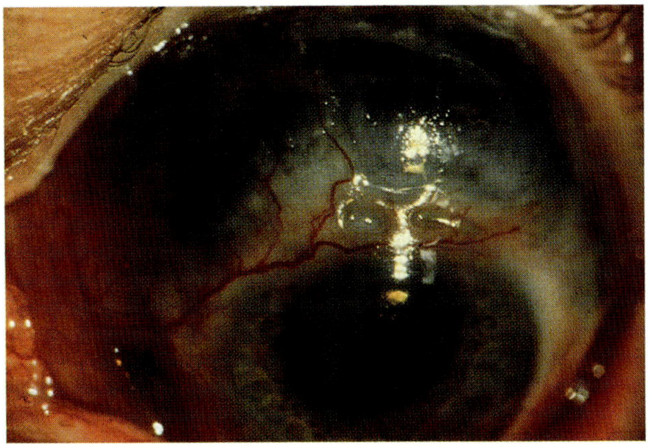

Rheumatoid arthritis, scleromalacia perforans.

Figure 5–49. Extensive superior scleral necrosis and uveal prolapse in severe case of scleromalacia perforans.

6

Tumors

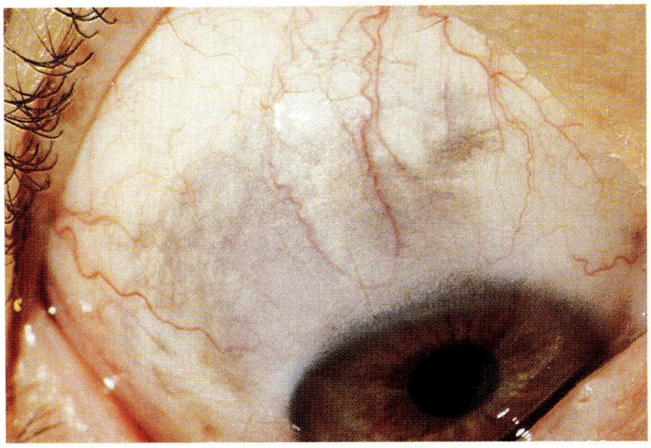

Benign acquired melanosis.

Figure 6–1. Ill-defined areas of melanotic stippling of the episclera in early case of benign acquired melanosis.

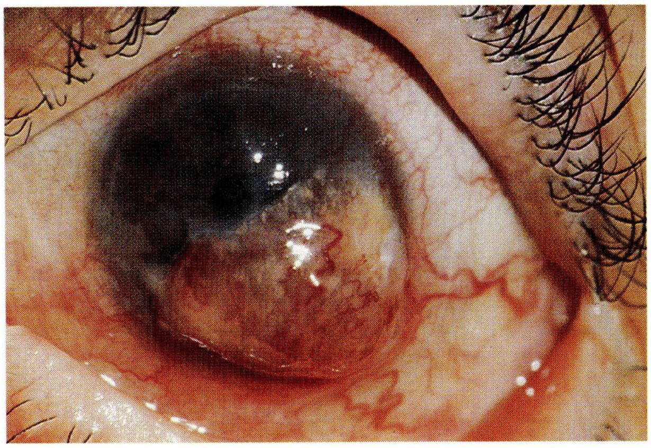

Melanoma.

Figure 6–2. A highly vascular, lightly pigmented epibulbar melanoma with corneal extension has arisen in an eye with extensive acquired melanosis.

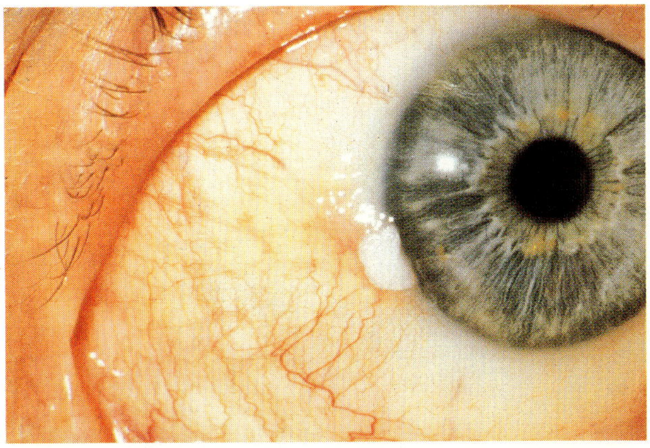

Squamous cell carcinoma in situ.

Figure 6–3. Focal hyperkeratotic plaque with minimal feeder vessels at the limbus was characterized pathologically by disorderly epithelial proliferation, keratinization, and increased mitotic activity.

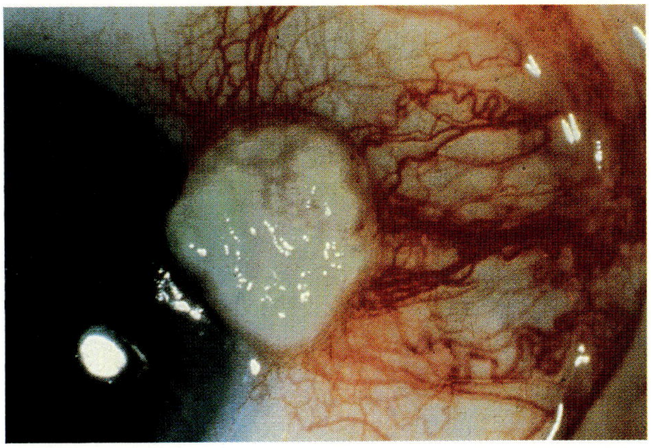

Squamous cell carcinoma.

Figure 6–4. A larger hyperkeratotic plaque with extensive feeder vessels (compare with Figure 6–3) characterized pathologically as a well-differentiated squamous cell carcinoma with subepithelial invasion of squamous cells.

Squamous cell carcinoma.

Figure 6–5. Rapidly growing, poorly differentiated squamous cell carcinoma with gelatinous papillary appearance and extension onto the cornea.

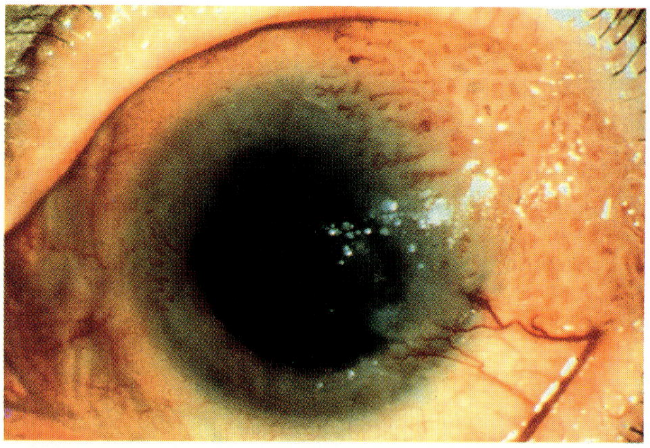

Squamous cell carcinoma, recurrent.

Figure 6–6. Extension of recurrent squamous cell carcinoma onto cornea as a raised, fleshy mass (arrow).

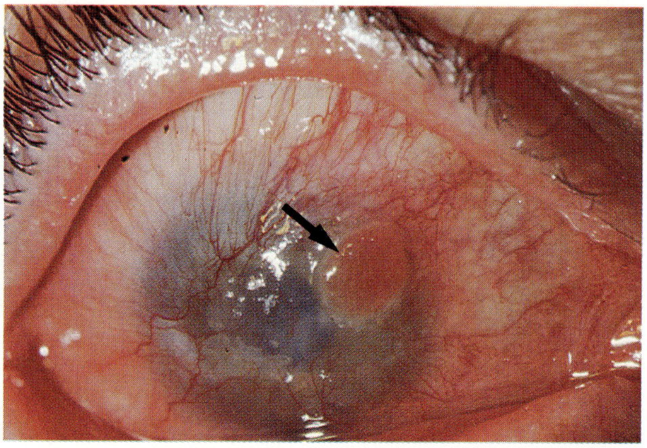

Squamous cell carcinoma, s/p resection without recurrence.

Figure 6–7. Same patient shown in Figure 6–6 five years later with no evidence of recurrent disease. Note persistence of corneal vascularity.

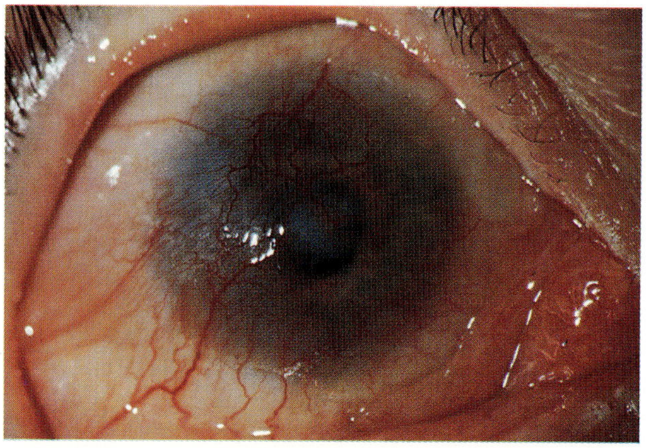

Sebaceous cell carcinoma.

Figure 6–8. Extensive corneal pannus in patient subsequently found to have a sebaceous gland carcinoma involving the lower lid, conjunctiva, and corneal epithelial surface.

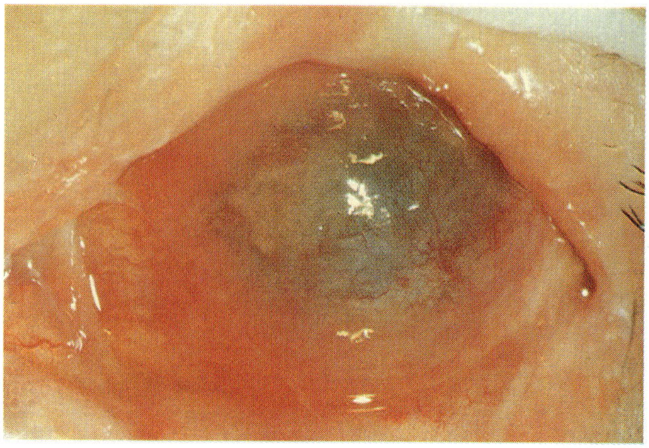

7

Congenital Anomalies

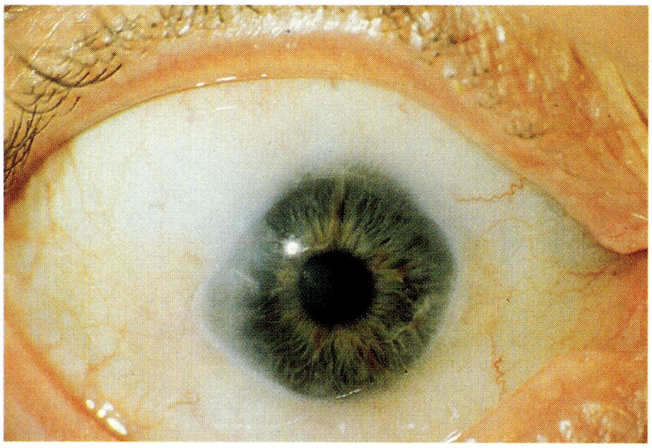

Microcornea.

Figure 7–1. Cornea 9.5 mm in diameter in young child with microcornea but no other associated ocular abnormalities.

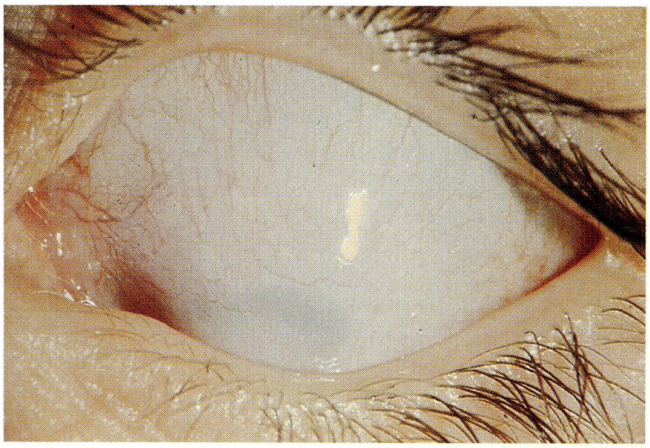

Sclerocornea.

Figure 7–2. Scleralization of the entire cornea is present in this eye, but the central cornea is slightly less opaque than the peripheral cornea. Note extension of superficial conjunctival and episcleral vessels onto the cornea without evidence of inflammation.

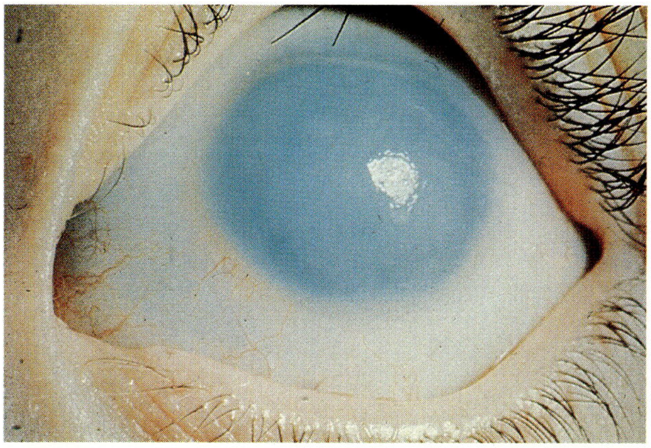

Congenital hereditary endothelial dystrophy, recessive form.

Figure 7–3. This severe corneal edema with marked thickening was present at birth.

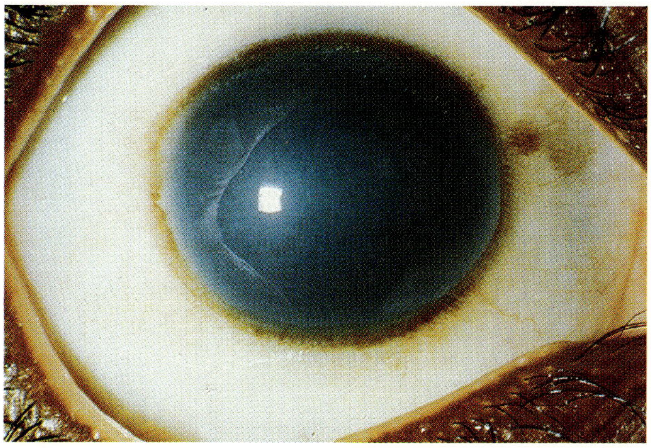

Congenital hereditary endothelial dystrophy, dominant form.

Figure 7–4. Milder corneal edema than seen in Figure 7–3 that became apparent during the first year of life. Iris details can still be faintly seen.

Kerectasia.

Figure 7–5. A large, unilateral bulging of the cornea with protrusion through the palpebral fissure was present at birth.

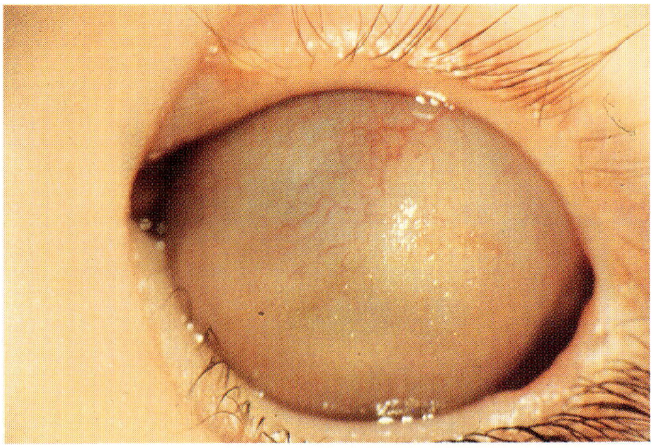

Anterior mesodermal dysgenesis, Peter's anomaly.

Figure 7–6. A dense, central corneal leukoma with adherent strands of iris with associated dense cataract is present in this variant of Peter's anomaly.

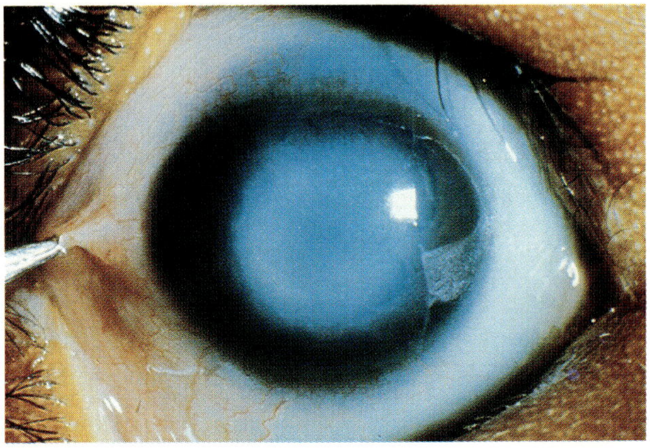

Anterior mesodermal dysgenesis, Axenfeld's anomaly.

Figure 7–7. Prominent iris processes are seen in association with exaggeration of the normal anterior border ring of Schwalbe's line (posterior embryotoxin, arrows).

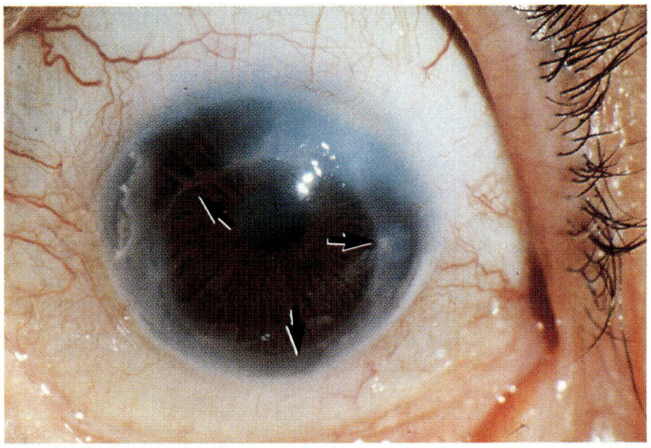

Goldenhar's syndrome, limbal dermoid.

Figure 7–8. Large white domelike mass (dermoid) unilaterally present in a child with preauricular appendages but no eyelid colobomas.

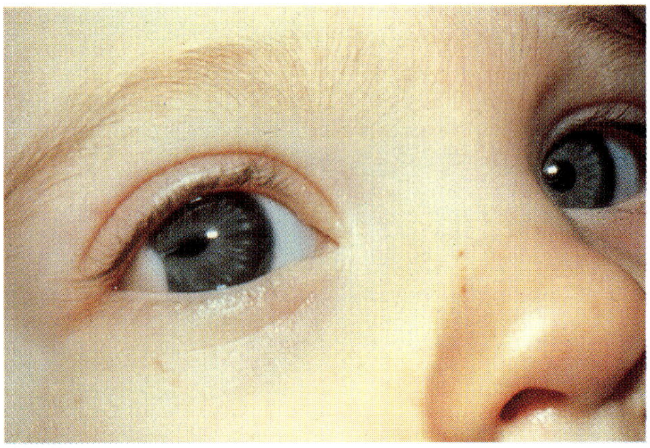

8

Trauma

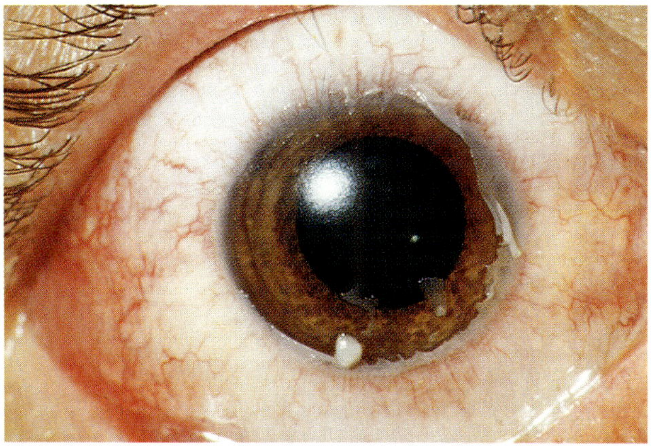

Chemical injury (mild, acute).

Figure 8–1. Total loss of corneal epithelium following battery explosion. Some denatured epithelium remains adherent to the globe at the limbus. The corneal stroma is clear, and the conjunctiva is still well vascularized.

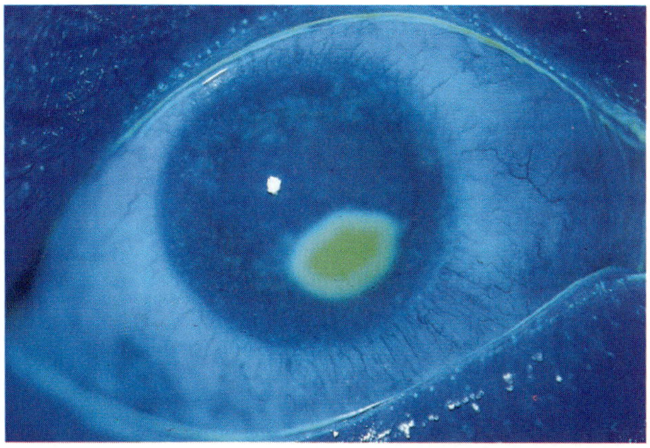

Chemical injury (mild, late).

Figure 8–2. Seven days later, the cornea shown in Figure 8–1 has 90 per cent reepithelialized with no significant complications.

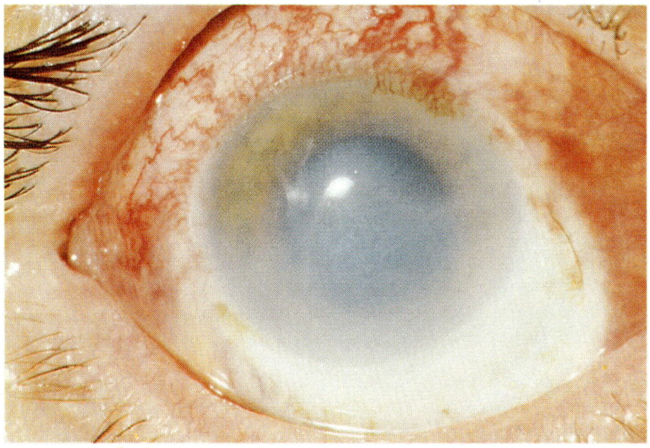

Chemical injury (severe, acute).

Figure 8–3. A severe alkali injury has resulted in a 100 per cent epithelial defect, loss of corneal clarity, and significant loss of vascularity of the inferonasal conjunctiva and sclera.

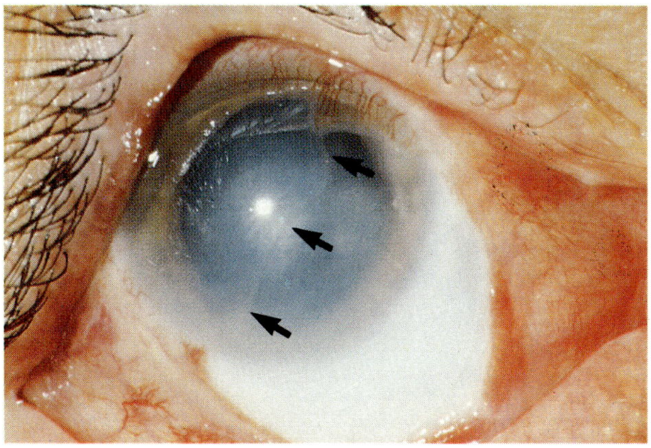

Chemical injury (severe, late).

Figure 8–4. Same patient shown in Figure 8–3, one month later. A persistent epithelial defect is present inferonasally (outlined with arrows), associated with the area of conjunctival and scleral necrosis and avascularity.

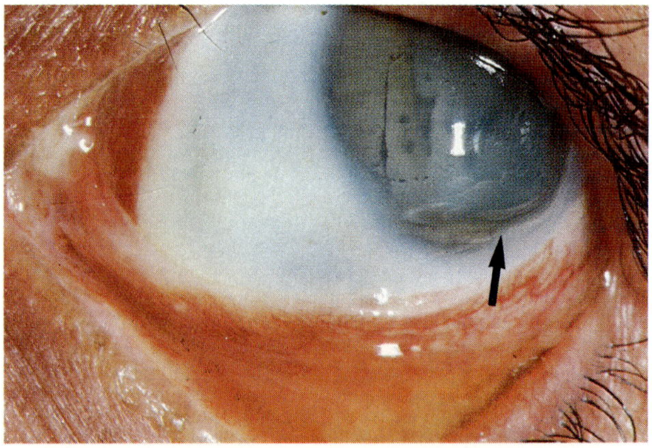

Chemical injury (late sequelae).

Figure 8–5. Two months following severe chemical injury, extensive conjunctival and scleral necrosis as well as a persistent epithelial defect and mature cataract are present. There is significant thinning of the inferior cornea (arrow).

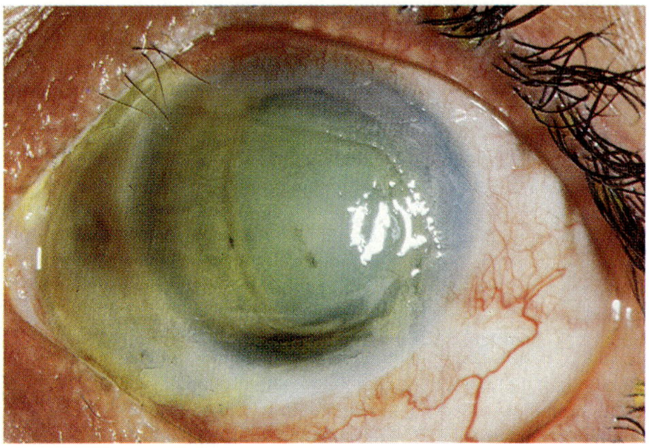

Chemical injury (late sequelae).

Figure 8–6. Same patient shown in Figure 8–5, seven days later. A 5 × 2 mm area of inferior cornea has perforated with prolapse of the iris and flattening of the anterior chamber.

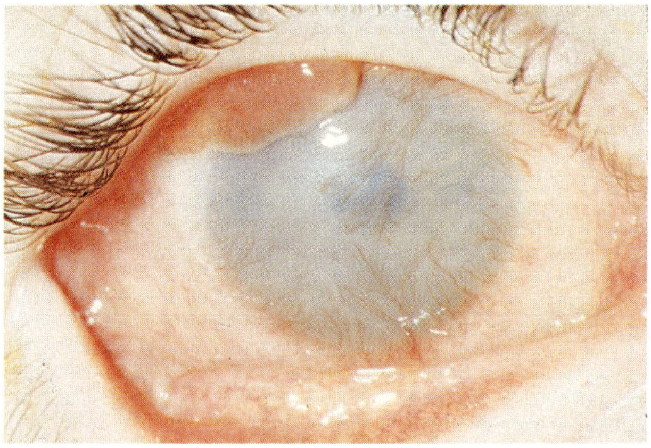

Chemical injury (late sequelae).

Figure 8–7. Superficial corneal vascularization with loss of corneal clarity six months following chemical injury.

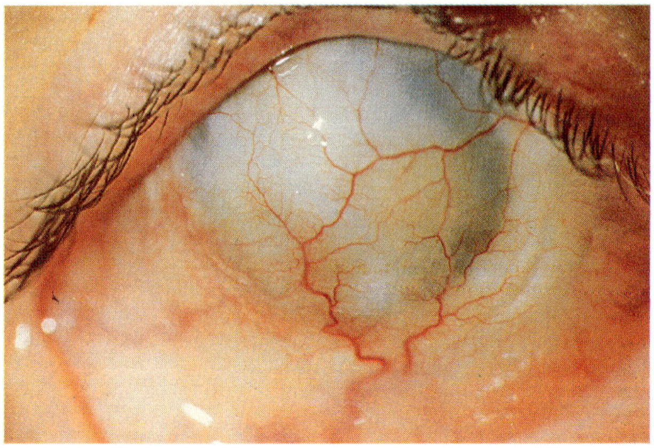

Chemical injury (late sequelae).

Figure 8–8. End stage corneal vascularization and cicatrization one year following severe chemical injury.

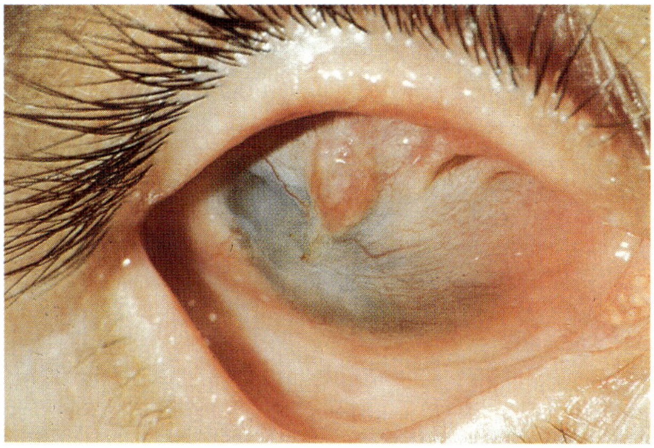

Chemical injury (late sequelae).

Figure 8–9. Extensive symblepharon of superior fornix to superior cornea, with associated corneal vasculature one year following acid injury. (From Brightbill, F.S. (ed.): Corneal Surgery. St. Louis, C.V. Mosby, 1986, p. 412.)

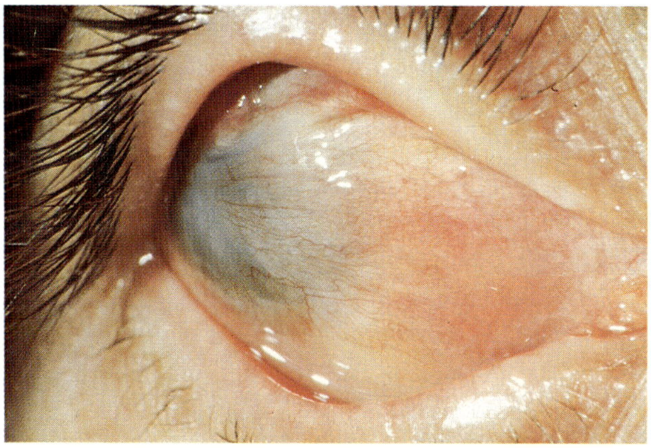

Chemical injury (late sequelae).

Figure 8–10. Lateral view of same patient shown in Figure 8–9.

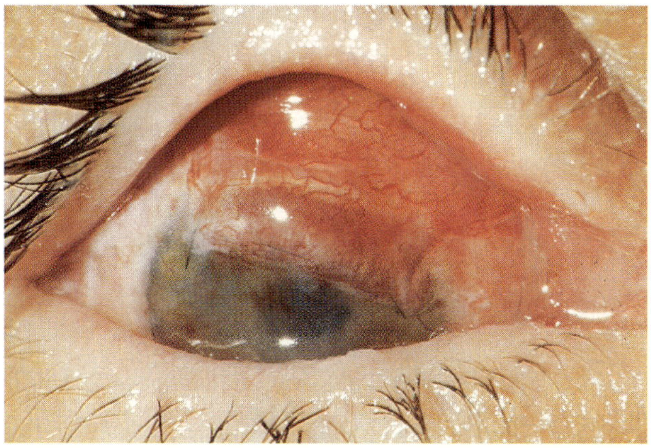

Chemical injury (s/p conjunctival transplant).

Figure 8–11. Same patient shown in Figure 8–9, one week following lysis of superior symblepharon, total superficial keratectomy, and superior limbic conjunctival transplantation from contralateral eye.

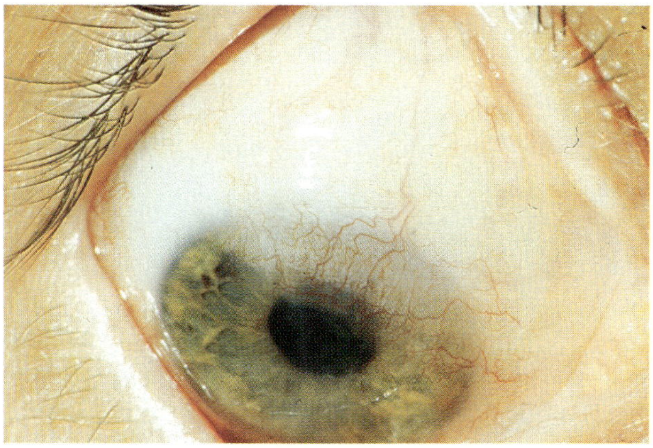

Chemical injury (s/p conjunctival transplant).

Figure 8–12. Same patient shown in Figure 8–9 one year later, demonstrating lack of recurrence of symblepharon, clearing of corneal pannus, and dramatically improved cosmesis and function. (From Brightbill, F.S. (ed.): Corneal Surgery. St. Louis, C.V. Mosby Co., 1986, p. 412.)

Chemical injury.

Figure 8–13. Severe corneal alkali injury with loss of corneal stromal clarity and persistent epithelial defect.

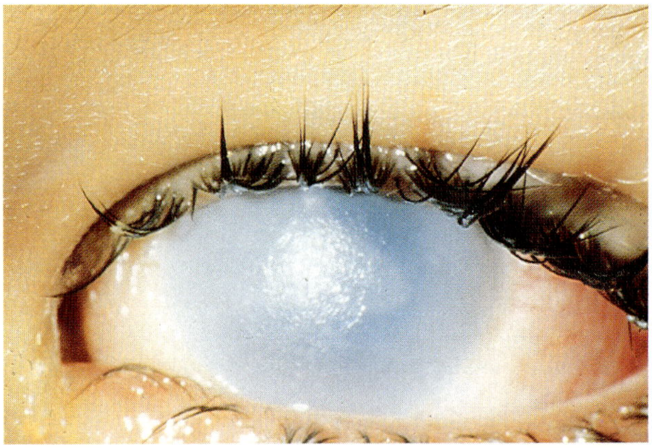

Chemical injury.

Figure 8–14. Same patient shown in Figure 8–13 following conjunctival transplantation. A 3 × 5 mm central epithelial defect persists.

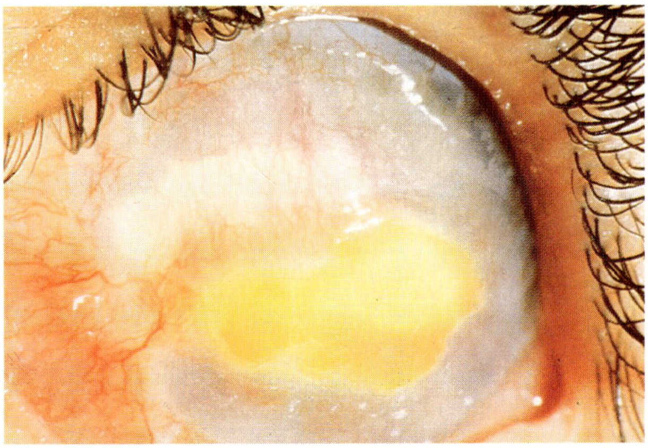

Chemical injury.

Figure 8–15. Same patient shown in Figure 8–13, six months following conjunctival transplant, with reepithelialized surface but persistent superficial stromal opacification and vascularization.

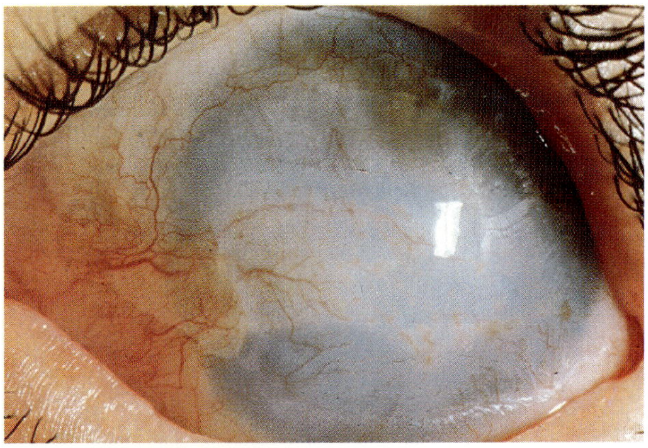

Chemical injury (s/p lamellar keratoplasty).

Figure 8–16. Same patient shown in Figure 8–13, two months following lamellar keratoplasty, which has reestablished corneal clarity. The epithelial surface is regular and clear.

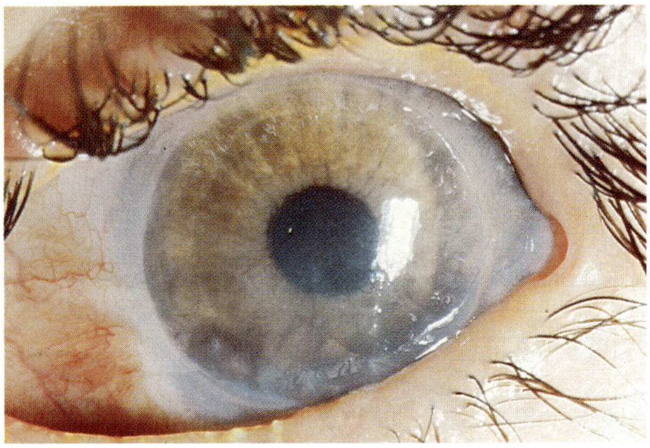

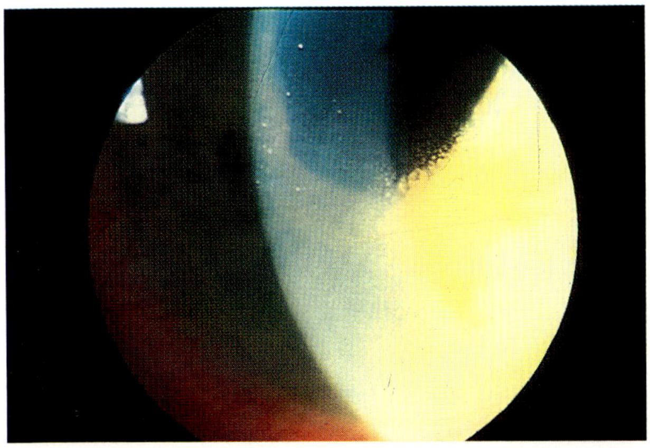

Contact lens trauma (hypoxia).

Figure 8–25. Advanced corneal microcystic edema associated with overwear of poorly fitted hard contact lens.

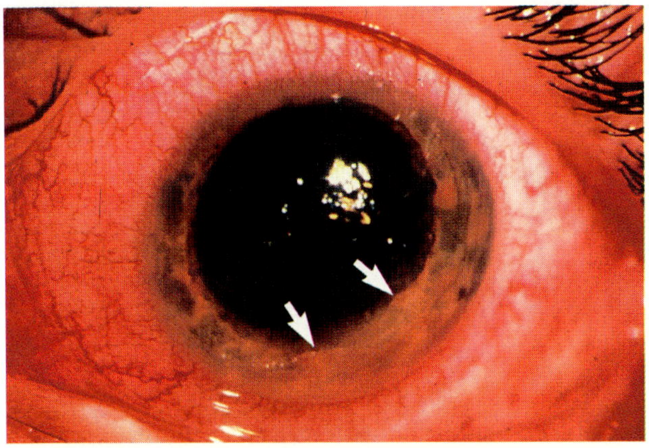

Contact lens trauma (hypoxia).

Figure 8–26. A well-defined (outlined by arrows) corneal epithelial defect can be seen beneath an extended wear soft contact lens.

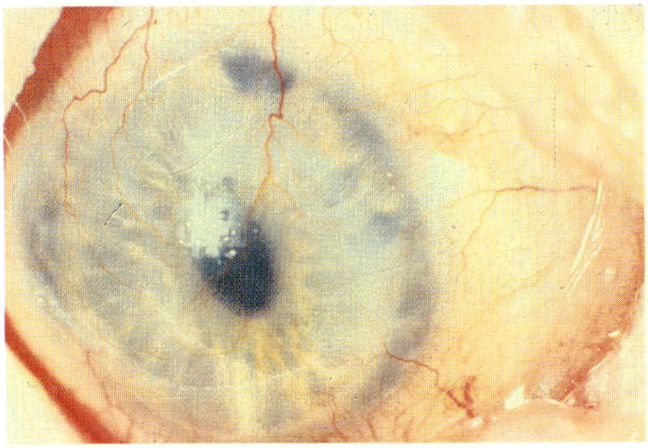

Contact lens trauma (hypoxia).

Figure 8–27. Extensive corneal vacularization has resulted from prolonged overwear of poorly fitted aphakic extended wear soft contact lens.

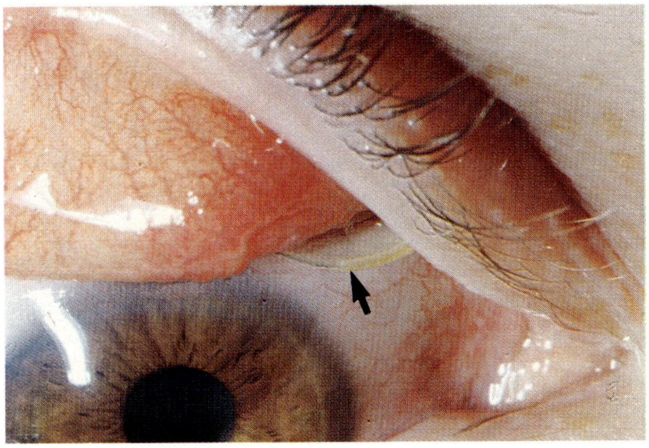

Contact lens trauma (giant papillary conjunctivitis).

Figure 8–28. Giant papillary conjunctivitis is present on the nasal aspect of the superior palpebral conjunctiva in association with trauma from a hard contact lens (arrow), which has been retained in the superior fornix for one year.

Surgical trauma (stripping of Descemet's membrane).

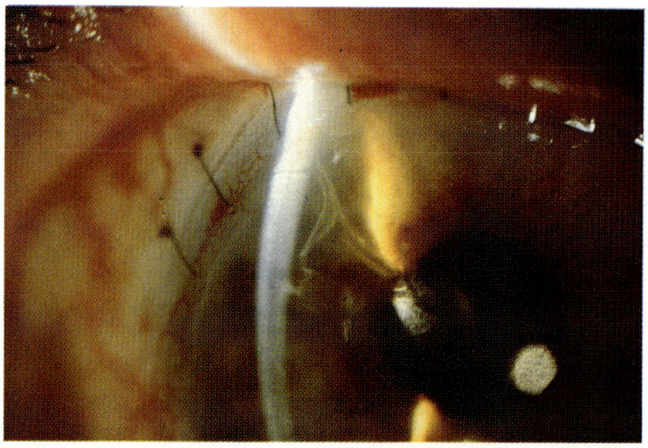

Figure 8–29. Inadvertent stripping of Descemet's membrane superiorly during cataract surgery has resulted in a "scroll-like" appearance of the loosened membrane. There are no associated functional abnormalities.

Surgical trauma (pseudophakic bullous keratopathy).

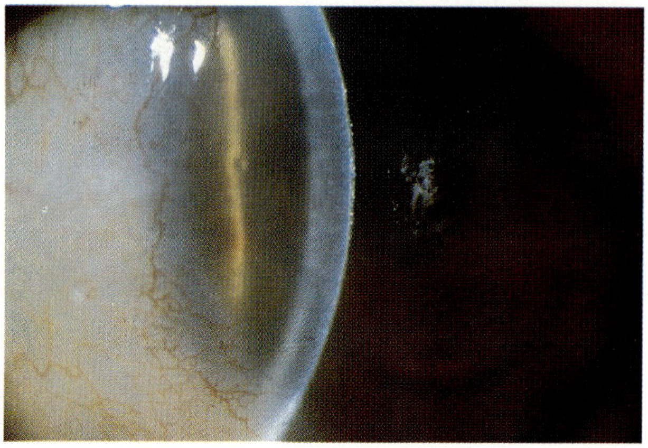

Figure 8–30. Six months following routine, uncomplicated intracapsular cataract extraction and implantation of anterior chamber intraocular lens, marked stromal and epithelial edema is seen.

Surgical trauma (endothelial blood staining).

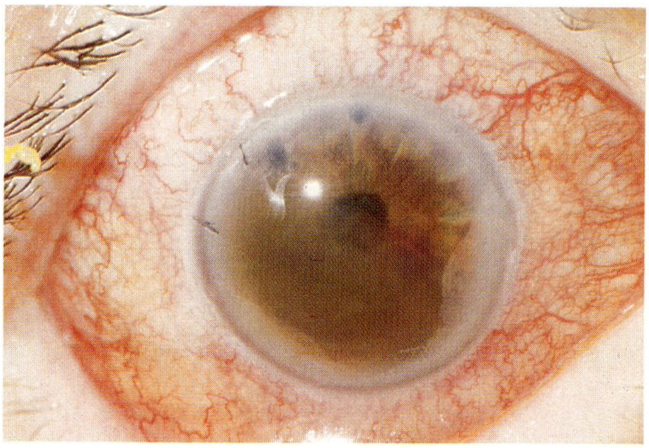

Figure 8–31. A postoperative hyphema with elevated intraocular pressure resulted in significant corneal endothelial blood staining, which is still present three months later.

Surgical trauma (intracorneal bleeding).

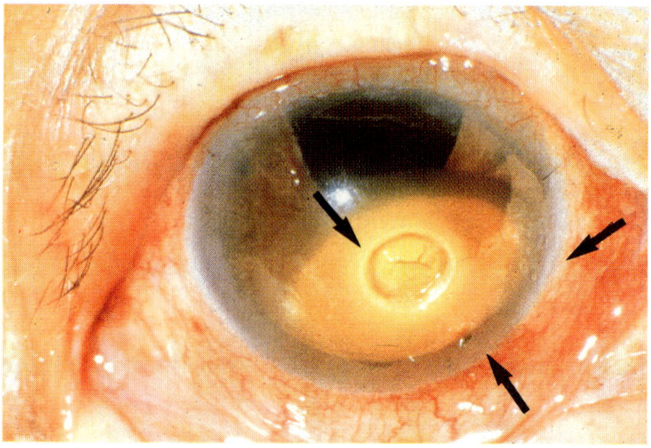

Figure 8–32. A large intracorneal hematoma (outlined by arrows) occurred following cyclodialysis. Two months later a central, 3 mm diameter area of corneal ulceration occurred. Descemet's membrane (with blood staining and a stellate perforation) is seen at the base of the area of ulceration.

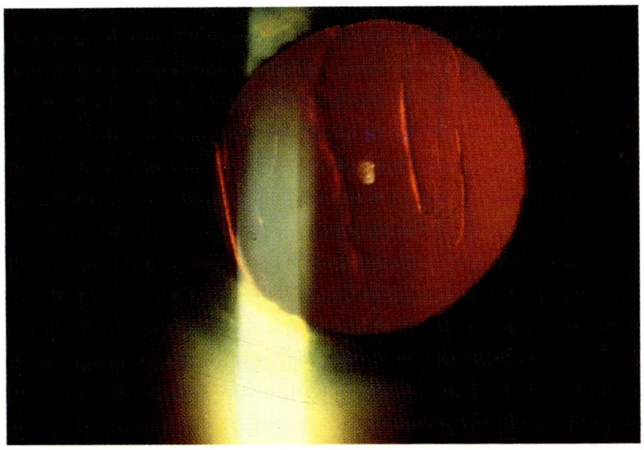

Forceps injury.

Figure 8–33. Vertically oriented linear breaks in Descemet's membrane resulting from forceps-related injury as seen with retroillumination. There is no associated corneal edema.

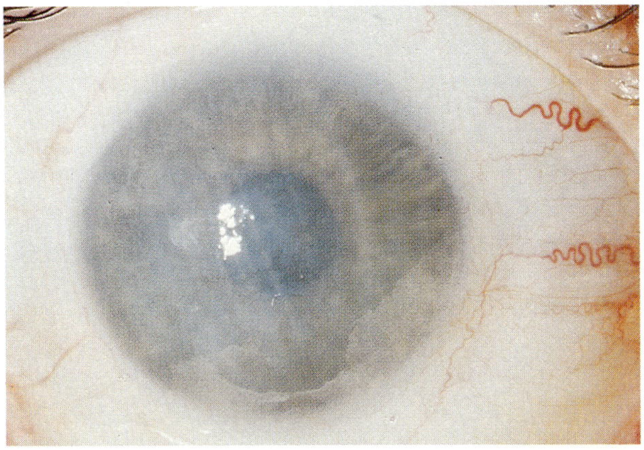

Forceps injury.

Figure 8–34. Severe corneal edema has resulted from endothelial dysfunction related to forceps injury. Linear streaks or breaks in Descemet's membrane can be easily seen.

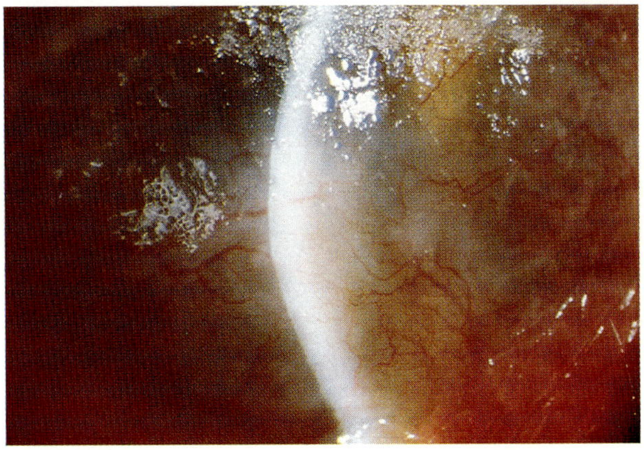

Radiation keratopathy.

Figure 8–35. Extensive corneal pannus following radiation of recurrent orbital basal cell carcinoma.

9

Surgical Complications

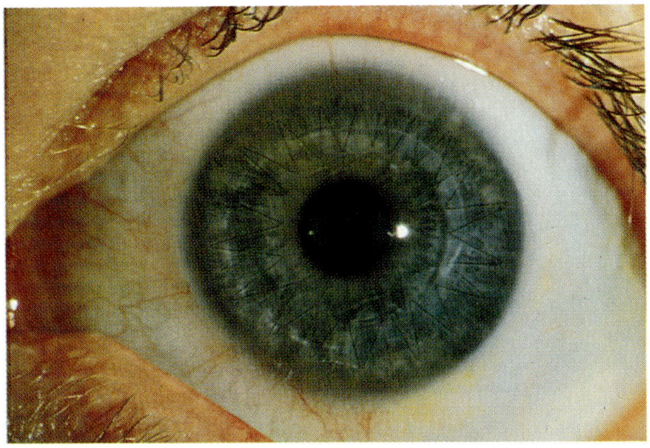

Penetrating keratoplasty.

Figure 9–1. Normal postoperative appearance of a penetrating keratoplasty performed for keratoconus. Wound is sutured with a single running 10–0 nylon suture.

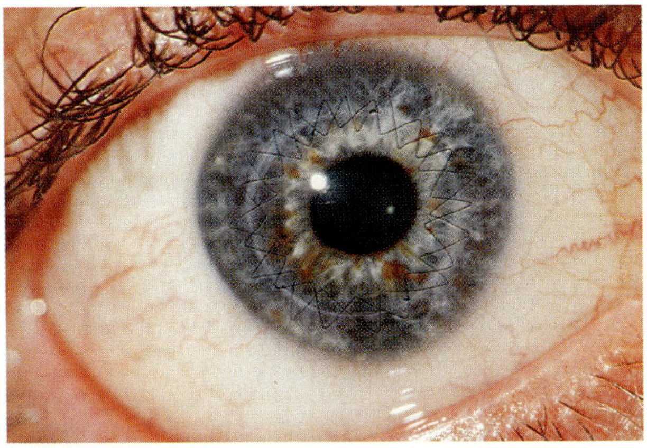

Penetrating keratoplasty.

Figure 9–2. Normal postoperative appearance of a penetrating keratoplasty performed for a central corneal scar. Wound is sutured with a double running 10–0 nylon suture.

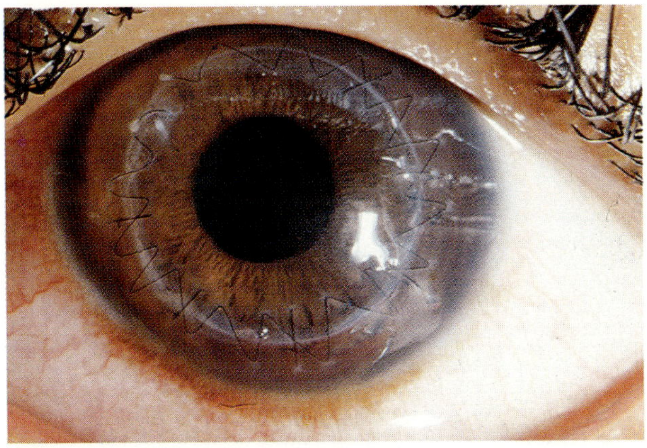

Corneal graft, loose sutures.

Figure 9–3. "Cheese wiring" of the running suture through the host cornea has resulted in loosening of the running suture at the 10:00 position with increased mucus accumulation and ocular inflammation. There is no wound leak or shallowing of anterior chamber.

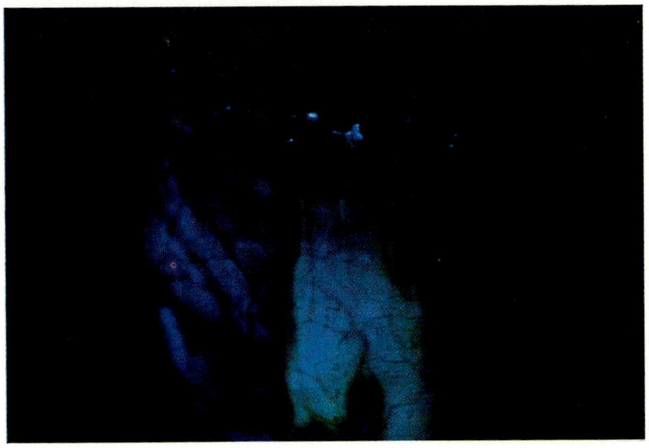

Corneal graft, wound leak.

Figure 9–4. Postoperative wound leak is demonstrated by Seidel's test. Fluorescein applied to the eye is diluted by aqueous in the area of the leak. (From Smolin, G., and Thoft, R. (eds.): The Cornea: Scientific Foundations and Clinical Practice. Boston, Little, Brown, and Co., 1983, p. 446.)

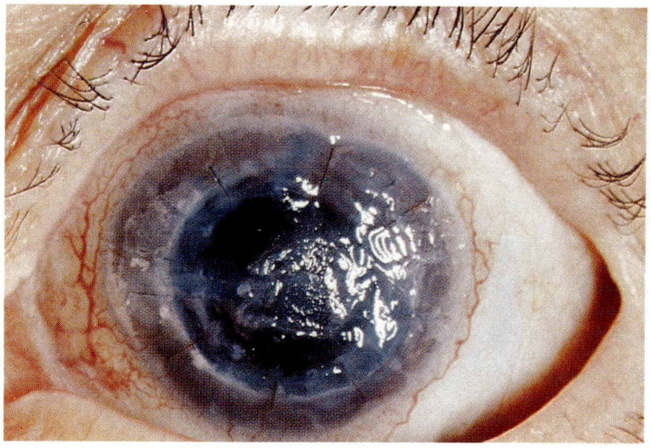

Corneal graft, band keratopathy.

Figure 9–5. Recurrent interpalpebral deposition of calcium in a six-month-old penetrating keratoplasty.

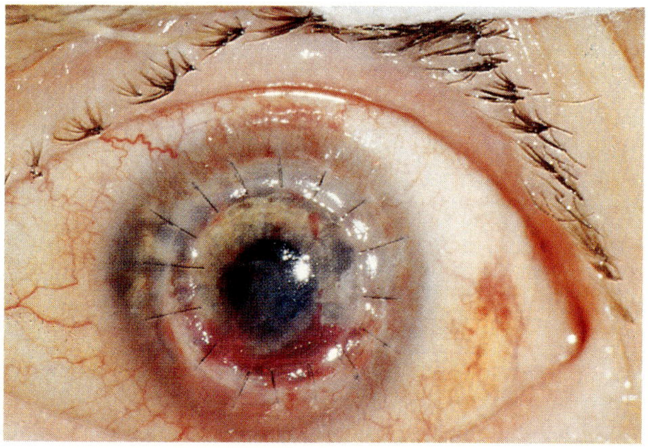

Corneal graft, peripheral anterior synechia.

Figure 9–6. Immediately following a penetrating keratoplasty for severe trophic ulceration due to herpes simplex virus keratitis, the anterior chamber has a marked fibrinoid response. There is a small postoperative hyphema and peripheral anterior synechia formation in the inferior angle.

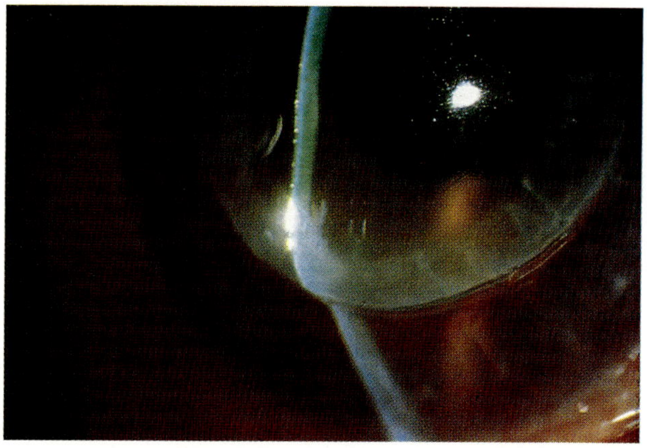

Corneal graft, wound dehiscence.

Figure 9–7. Marked anterior bulge of the corneal graft is seen following suture removal.

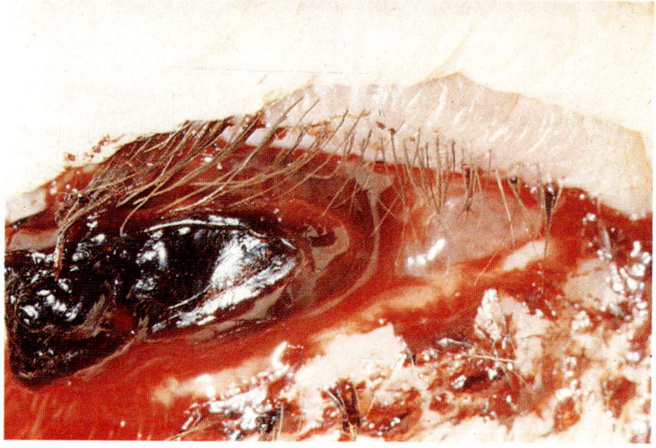

Corneal graft, ruptured globe.

Figure 9–8. Blunt trauma to the globe three months after penetrating keratoplasty has resulted in complete dehiscence of the corneal graft and expulsion of intraocular contents.

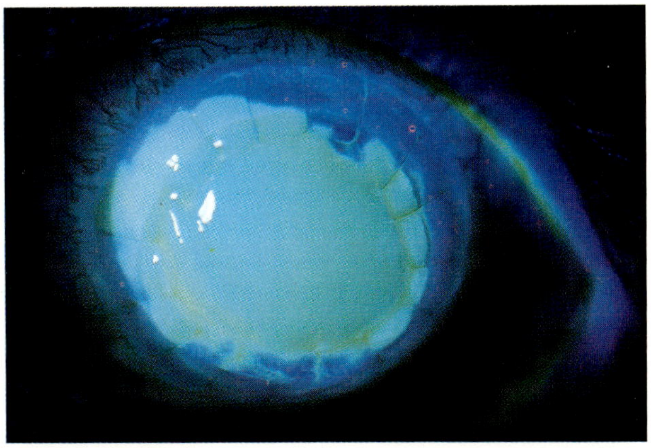

Corneal graft, persistent epithelial defect.

Figure 9–9. Tectonic graft performed for unilateral Mooren's ulcer has had persistent epithelial defect for several months despite intensive lubrication, contact lens, tarsorrhaphy, and epidermal growth factor therapy.

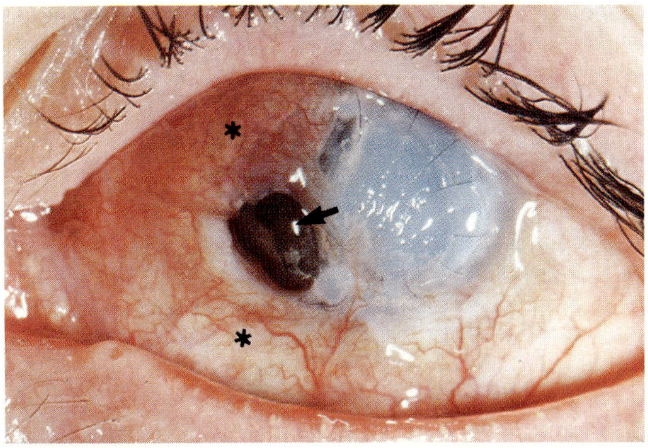

Corneal graft, corneal perforation.

Figure 9–10. Despite conjunctival transplantation (asterisks), the cornea shown in Figure 9–9 has had sterile ulceration and extensive perforation (arrow) with iris prolapse. Note severe loss of clarity of remaining graft.

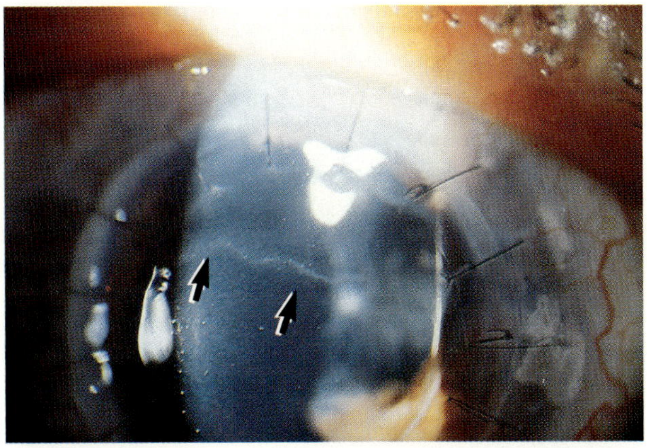

Corneal graft, epithelial rejection.

Figure 9–11. Well-defined epithelial rejection line (outlined by arrows) separates normal corneal epithelium (inferiorly) from involved area superiorly. Note minimal effect on epithelial clarity.

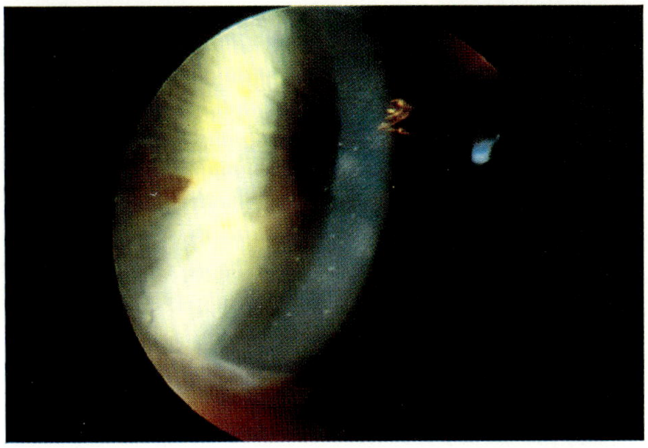

Corneal graft, epithelial rejection.

Figure 9–12. Epithelial rejection in this case is manifested by subepithelial deposits similar to those seen in epidemic keratoconjunctivitis (see Figure 3–30). (From Smolin, G., and Thoft, R. (eds.): The Cornea: Scientific Foundations and Clinical Practice. Boston, Little, Brown, and Co., 1983, p. 449.)

Corneal graft, endothelial rejection.

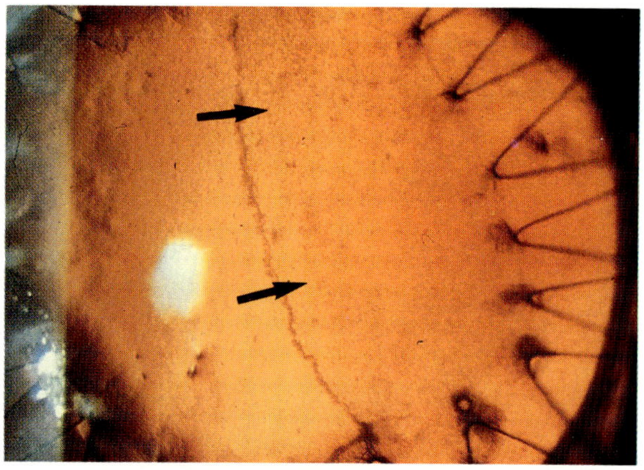

Figure 9–13. Classic endothelial rejection line (arrows) seen in retroillumination. Keratic precipitates can be seen on the endothelium to the right of the rejection line. (From Brightbill, F.S. (ed.): Corneal Surgery. St. Louis, C.V. Mosby Co., 1986, p. 381.)

Corneal graft, endothelial rejection.

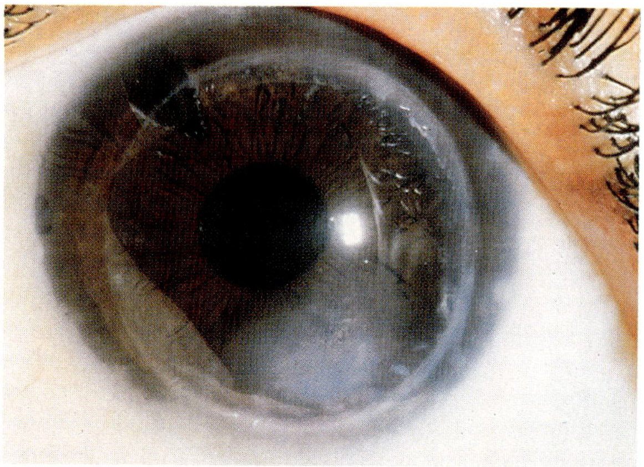

Figure 9–14. Following resolution of the endothelial rejection episode in this cornea, irreversible corneal edema persists. Because the visual axis was spared, visual acuity remains good.

Corneal graft, endothelial rejection.

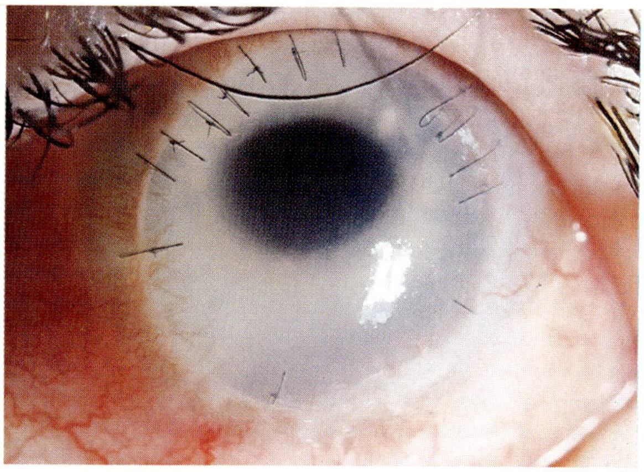

Figure 9–15. In this case, endothelial rejection is characterized by extensive, diffuse keratic precipitates, corneal edema, and migration of deep stromal vessels into the graft. This episode occurred three weeks following penetrating keratoplasty for extensive fungal keratitis with perforation.

Corneal graft, endothelial rejection.

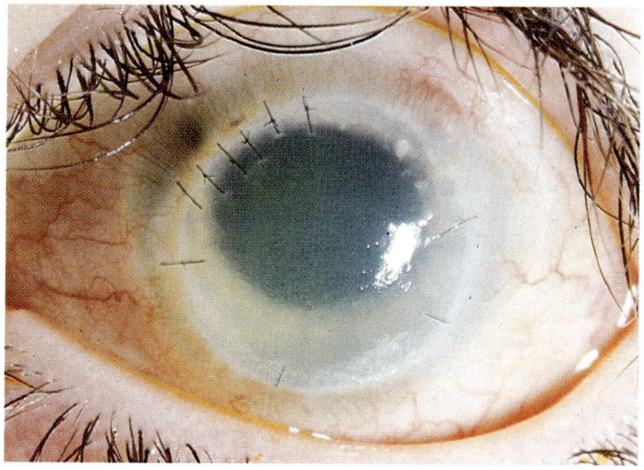

Figure 9–16. Following control of the inflammation in the cornea shown in Figure 9–15, microcystic epithelial edema persists. The keratic precipitates have resolved, and vascularization of the donor cornea has been arrested.

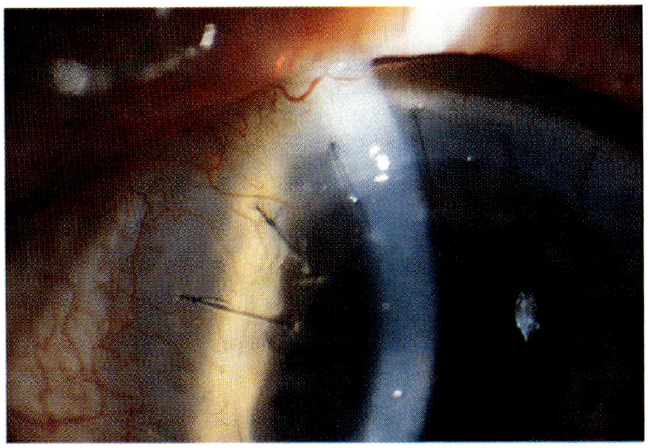

Corneal graft, early vascularization.

Figure 9–17. A loose interrupted suture has resulted in vascularization extending to the graft-host junction and precipitated an early rejection episode.

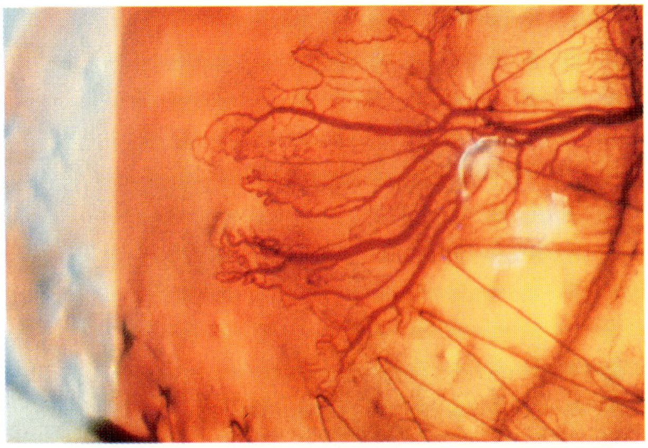

Corneal graft, advanced vascularization.

Figure 9–18. Extensive mid-stromal vascularization of the donor cornea is demonstrated by retroillumination.

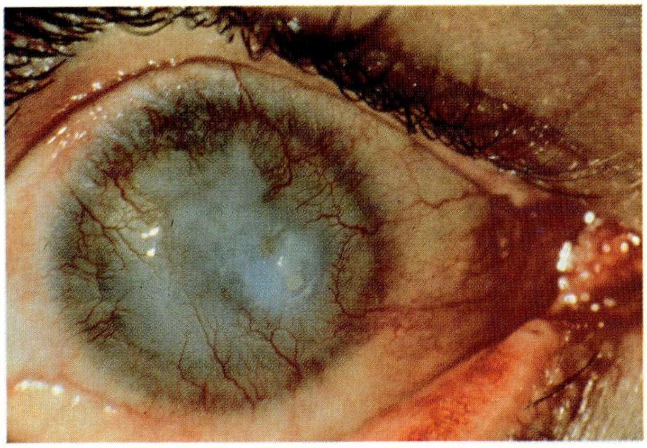

Corneal graft failure.

Figure 9–19. Extensive vascularization and loss of clarity has occurred in this graft performed for extensive chemical injury.

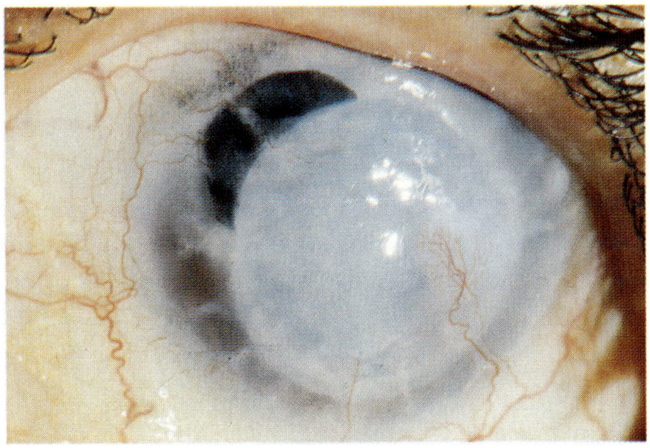

Corneal graft failure.

Figure 9–20. Vascularization of this eccentrically placed graft in a keratoconic eye has resulted in loss of clarity and failure. Note contrasting clarity of the recipient cornea.

Corneal graft, fungal keratitis.

Figure 9–21. A deep stroma infiltrate along the path of an interrupted suture subsequently proved to harbor *Candida albicans*.

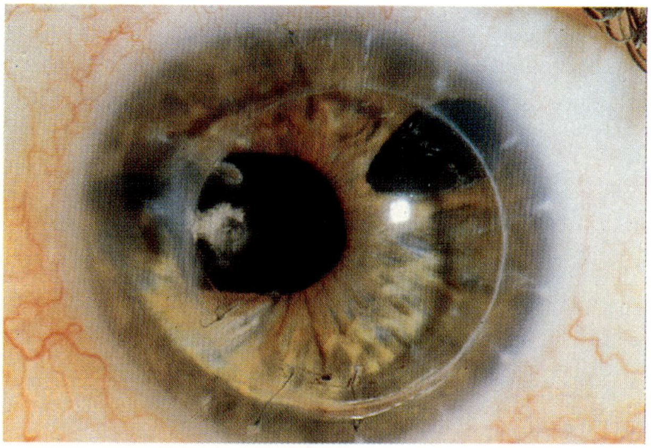

Corneal graft, recurrent herpes simplex keratitis.

Figure 9–22. Classic herpetic dendritic epithelial keratitis on a recent penetrating keratoplasty receiving topical steriods but no antivirals.

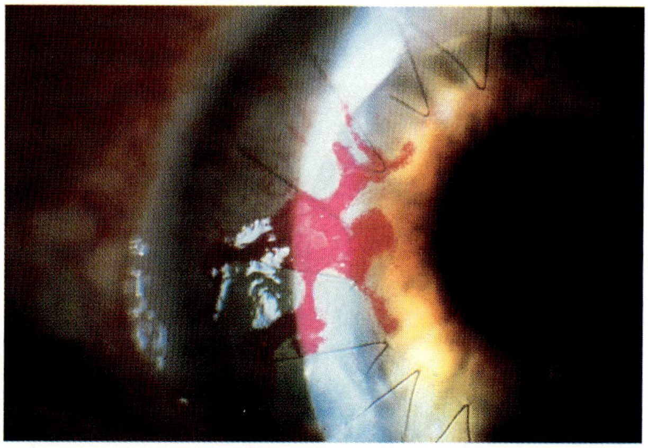

Corneal graft, *Pseudomonas* keratitis.

Figure 9–23. Within 48 hours, a small infiltrate at the graft-host junction has extended intraocularly and into adjacent limbus and sclera, ultimately resulting in the loss of the eye.

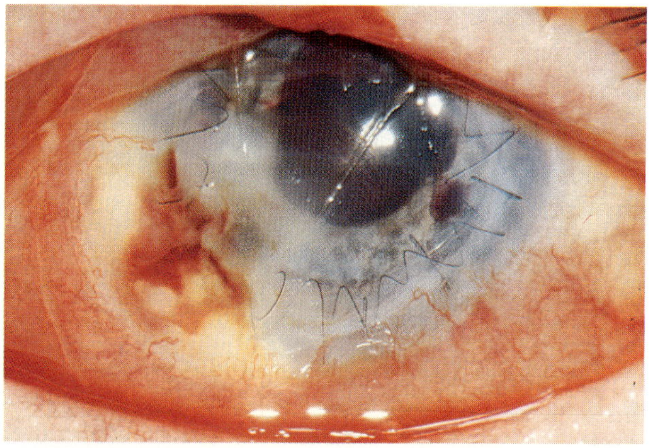

Corneal graft, endophthalmitis.

Figure 9–24. Thirty-six hours following uncomplicated penetrating keratoplasty, extensive panophthalmitis due to B-hemolytic *Streptococcus* resulted in complete destruction of the scleral coat of the eye, expulsive hemorrhage with loss of intraocular contents, and complete dehiscence of the graft, which has been dislocated to the lateral canthus. The donor button was culture-positive for the organism.

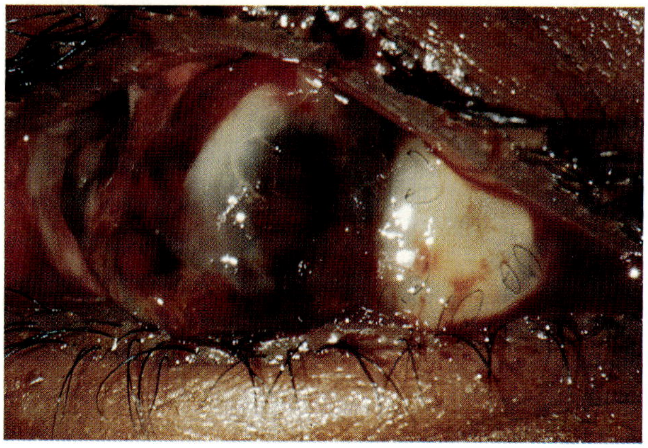

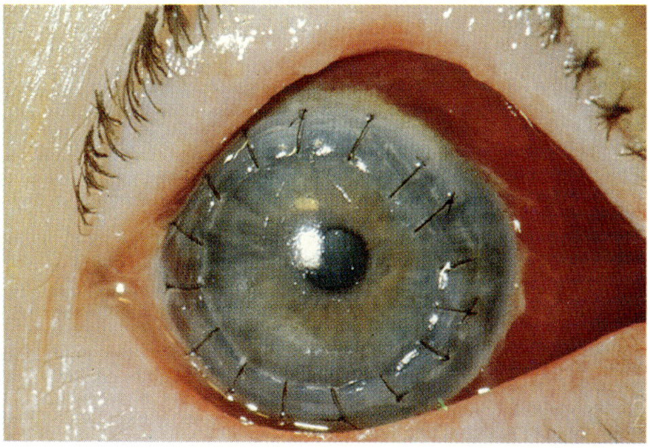

Lamellar keratoplasty.

Figure 9–25. Early postoperative appearance of lamellar graft performed for Reis-Buckler dystrophy.

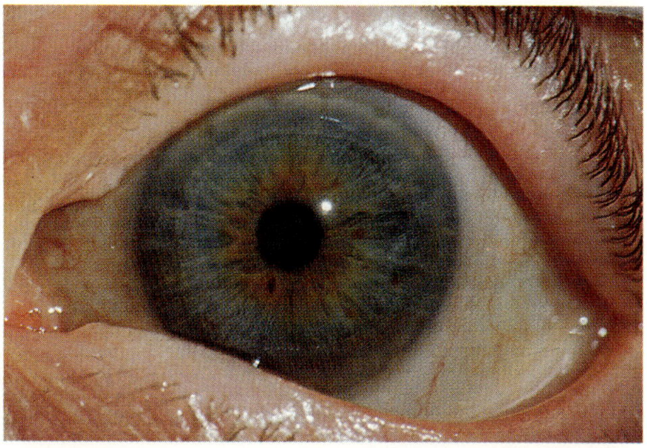

Lamellar keratoplasty.

Figure 9–26. Six years later, the patient shown in Figure 9–25 has corneal clarity similar to that seen with a penetrating keratoplasty (Figures 9–1 and 9–2).

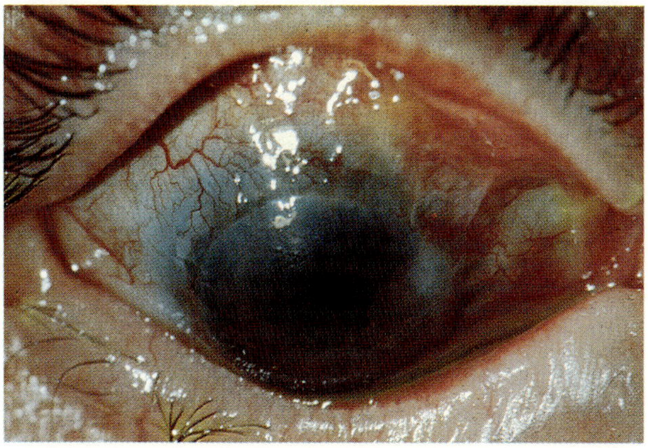

Lamellar keratoplasty (vascularization).

Figure 9–27. In this early, clear lamellar keratoplasty, vascularization of the graft-host interface can already be seen.

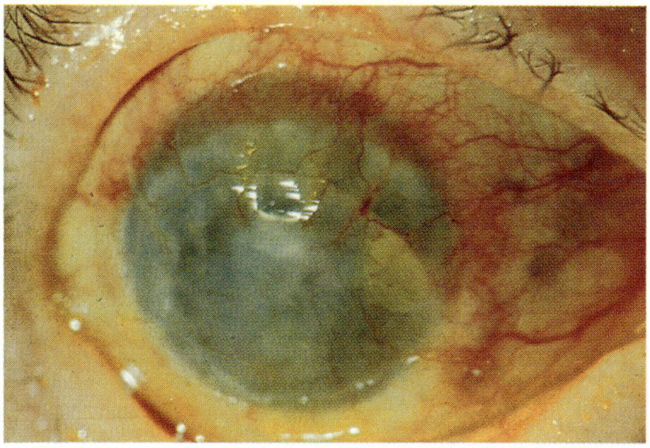

Lamellar keratoplasty (vascularization).

Figure 9–28. Complete opacification and scarring of the button has followed advanced vascularization of the graft-host interface.

Tectonic lamellar keratoplasty (preoperative).

Figure 9–29. Advanced peripheral corneal ulcerative keratitis due to Mooren's ulceration has resulted in corneal perforation and flat anterior chamber. (From DeLuise, V.P., and Tabbara, K.F. (ed.): International Ophthalmology Clinics: Peripheral Corneal Diseases, volume 26. Boston, Little, Brown, and Co., 1986, p. 156.)

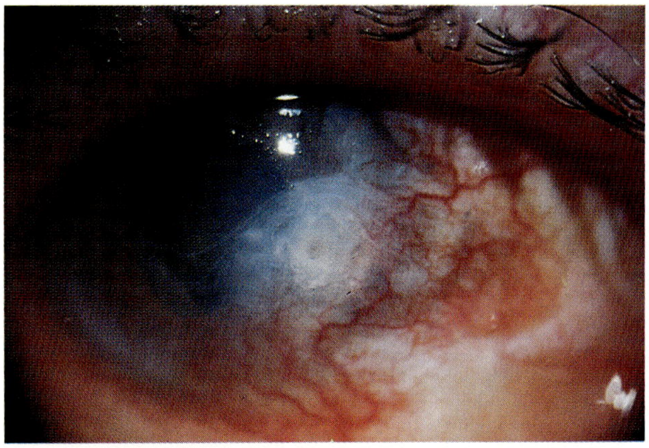

Tectonic lamellar keratoplasty (postoperative).

Figure 9–30. Same patient shown in Figure 9–29, following corneoscleral lamellar tectonic graft. (From DeLuise, V.P., and Tabbara, K.F. (ed.): International Ophthalmology Clinics: Peripheral Corneal Disease, volume 26. Boston, Little, Brown, and Co., 1986, p. 156.)

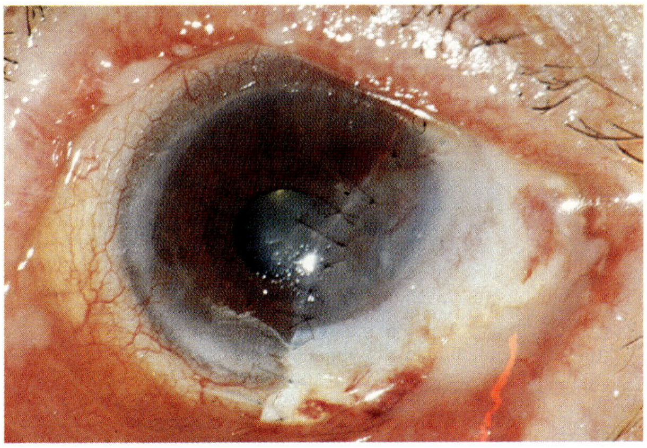

Epikeratoplasty (aphakic, early postoperative appearance).

Figure 9–31. One-week postoperative appearance of aphakic keratoplasty in a traumatically monocularly aphakic eye. Two sutures (10:30, 1:30) have already been removed. Reepithelialization is complete.

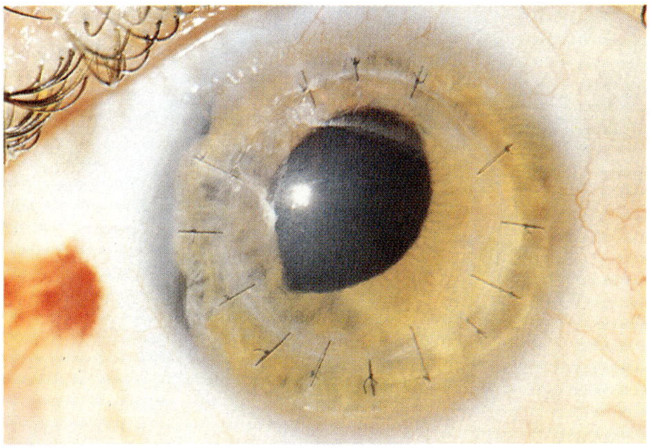

Epikeratoplasty (aphakic, late postoperative appearance).

Figure 9–32. Three months following aphakic epikeratoplasty, and one month following removal of final sutures, epikeratoplasty button is crystal clear with no loss of clarity at the graft-host interface.

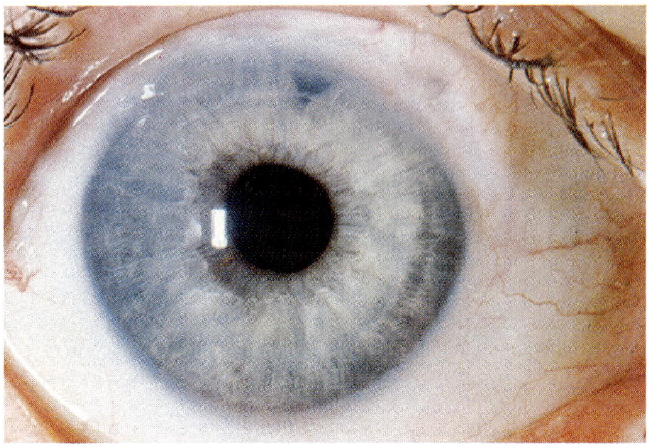

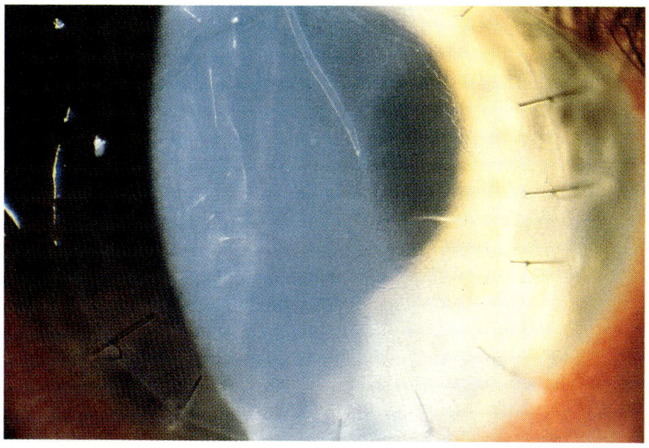

Epikeratoplasty (keratoconus, early postoperative appearance).

Figure 9–33. Following epikeratoplasty for keratoconus, extensive flattening of the cornea results in extensive folding in host Descemet's membrane.

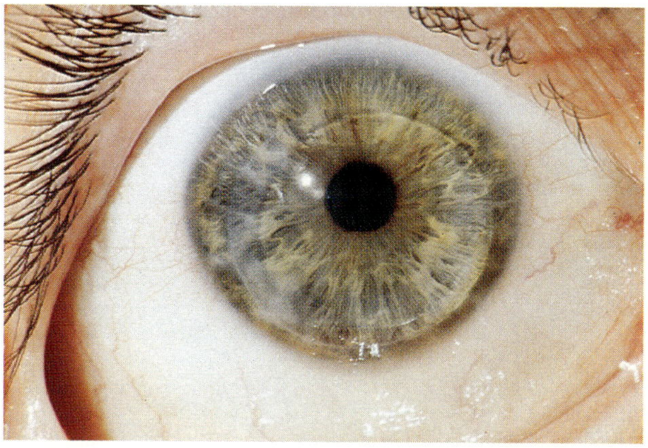

Epikeratoplasty (keratoconus, late postoperative appearance).

Figure 9–34. Eight months later, the cornea shown in Figure 9–33 has no residual folds in Descemet's membrane. As in Figure 9–32, the graft is crystal clear and there are no interface opacities.

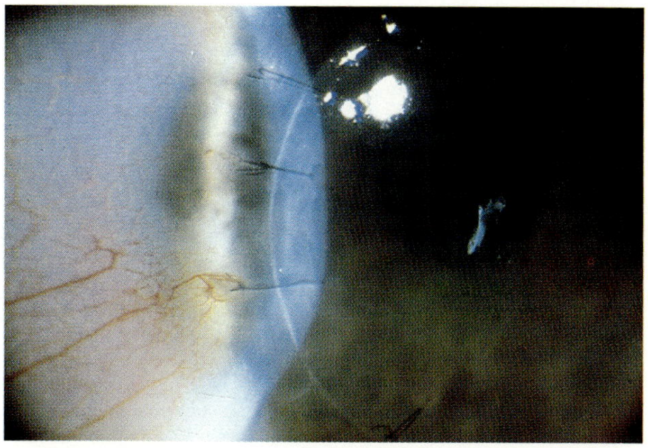

Epikeratoplasty, suture vascularization.

Figure 9–35. Vascularization and loosening of corneal suture due to inadequate postoperative topical steroid therapy.

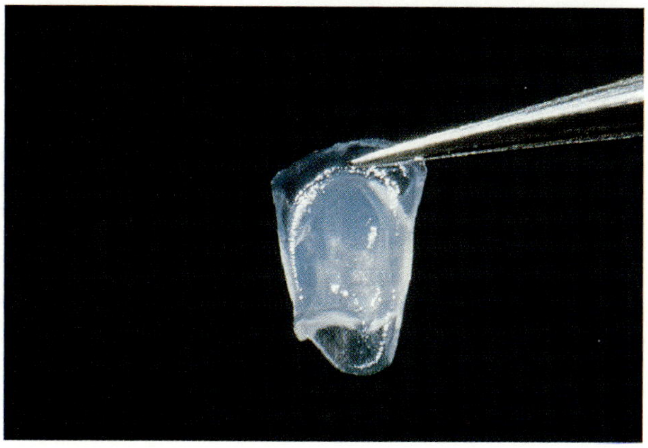

Epikeratoplasty, retrolenticular membrane.

Figure 9–36. Two weeks following epikeratoplasty, a dense retrolenticular membrane resulted in complete loss of clarity. Following removal, a dense, opaque plaque can be seen adherent to the posterior surface of the lenticule.

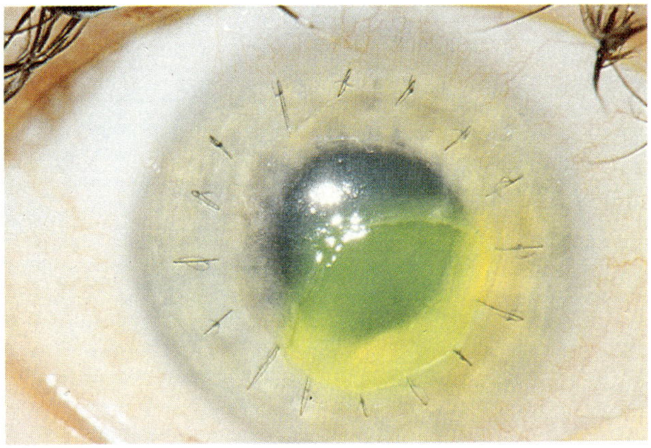

Epikeratoplasty, persistent epithelial defect.

Figure 9–37. Following postoperative reepithelialization, a traumatic abrasion (mascara brush) failed to heal despite intensive medical therapy.

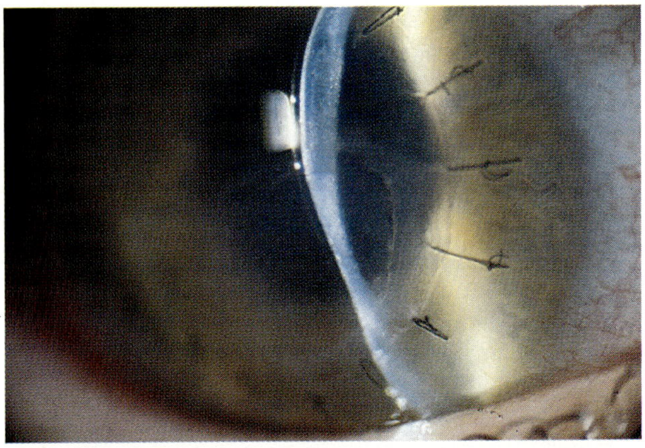

Epikeratoplasty, sterile ulceration.

Figure 9–38. The same patient shown in Figure 9–37, two weeks later. The epithelial defect has remained unchanged, but dissolution of the underlying stroma has begun.

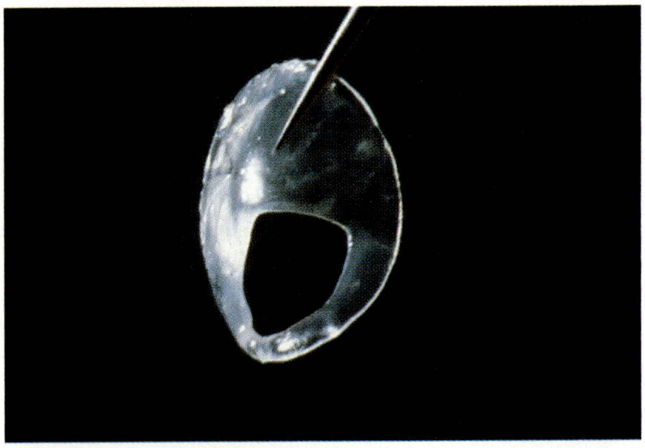

Epikeratoplasty, sterile ulceration.

Figure 9–39. Appearance of epikeratoplasty lenticule shown in Figure 9–38, at the time of removal. Note complete loss of stroma in the distribution of the persistent epithelial defect. (From Frangieh, G.H., Kenyon, K.R., Wagoner, M.D., et al.: Epithelial abnormalities and sterile stromal ulceration in epikeratoplasty grafts. Ophthalmology 95:213–227, 1988.)

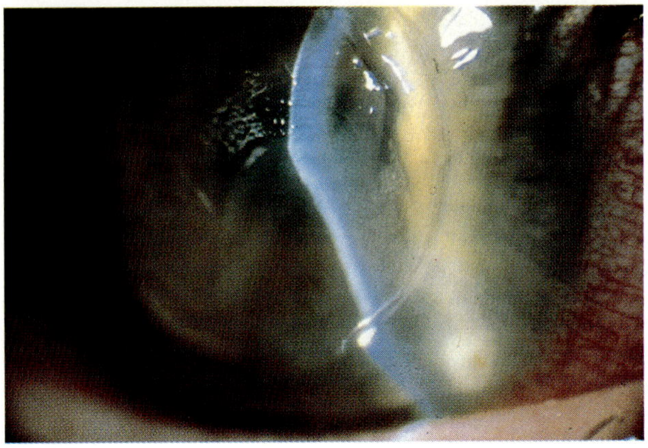

Epikeratoplasty, sterile ulceration of recipient cornea.

Figure 9–40. Same patient shown in Figures 9–37 and 9–38, following removal of epikeratoplasty lenticule. Extensive sterile ulceration of the patient's own cornea has resulted in 50 per cent loss of corneal stroma in the distribution of the epikeratoplasty lenticule epithelial defect. (From Frangieh, G.H., Kenyon, K.R., Wagoner, M.D., et al.: Epithelial abnormalities and sterile stromal ulceration in epikeratoplasty grafts. Ophthalmology 95:213–227, 1988.)

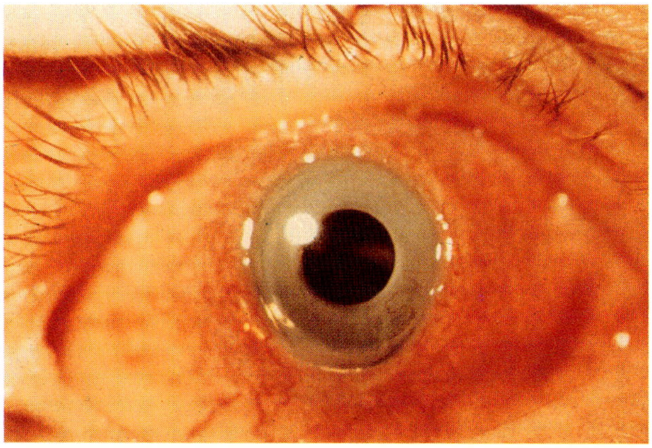

Keratoprosthesis, early postoperative appearance.

Figure 9–41. Keratoprosthesis is securely in place with no evidence of dehiscence immediately postoperatively.

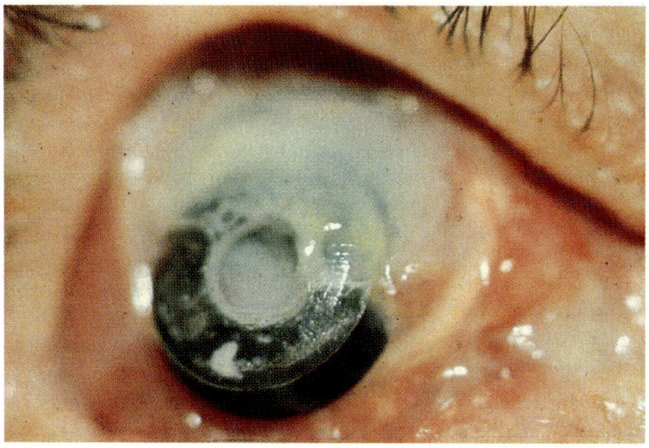

Keratoprosthesis, late postoperative appearance.

Figure 9–42. Characteristic late appearance of keratoprosthesis with extrusion of implant associated with necrosis of adjacent host tissue.

Index